Up The Creek With a Paddle

Beat MS and Many Autoimmune Disorders with Low Dose Naltrexone (LDN)

Mary Anne Boyle Bradley

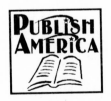

PublishAmerica
Baltimore

First printing

ISBN: 1-4137-6599-8
PUBLISHED BY PUBLISHAMERICA, LLLP
www.publishamerica.com
Baltimore

Printed in the United States of America

Dedicated To Rosemary Konde

It takes a minute to find a special person,
an hour to appreciate them,
a day to love them,
but then an entire life to forget them.

Thanks so much for your time!

Dear Dr. Flanzman

I wish there were more
doctors like you!

Thank You

Mary A Bradley

"Books are never out of humor or pride,
never envious or jealous,
they answer all questions with readiness,
they teach us how to live,
and how to die;
they dispel melancholy by their mirth,
and amuse by their wit,
they prepare the soul to suffer everything and desire nothing;
they introduce us to ourselves."

Holbrook Jackson

Introduction

I have a story I want all of Ireland, and indeed the world, to hear. I tried to entice a popular talk show host in Ireland, Pat Kenny, to tell it and I honestly think that he will do some sort of a show on this topic someday. I also wrote to Oprah and I firmly believe that she too will air something about it someday. In the meantime, I have decided to write the whole thing down.

Actually, I tried to entice numerous celebrities to carry the torch, but for now it seems that they are not brave enough to take a leap of faith and just run with it. I cannot blame them because it is difficult to believe.

Keith Finnegan, to his credit, *did* actually bite the bullet and give me a window on his radio show on Galway Bay FM on April 30th 2004. Afterwards I was happy enough, but I cannot help but feel that I should have said more. The story is just so big. It is my hope that the hero of this story, Dr. Bernard Bihari, receives full recognition, perhaps even a Nobel Prize one day. However, in the grand scheme of things, TV, radio and prizes matter very little.

People matter. People really count. Every single person counts, and that is why I want to tell my story. I will start at the beginning.

Chapter 1

I was born in Cook County Hospital in Chicago on June 11th 1971. My parents, Maureen and Vincent Boyle, are originally from Arranmore Island off the coast of Donegal, Ireland. I am their forth child out of five and their only daughter. My three older brothers are named Pat, Phil and Vince and a year separates them all. There are two years between Vince and me. My parents aptly named me Mary Anne after my maternal grandmother. Aptly, because even I can see the resemblance.

In many ways I have been blessed with two sets of parents. I rarely say Mom and Dad. Instead, I generally say Mom, Dad, Annie and Neilus. Annie and Neilus Bonner are my aunt and uncle, and they live on Arranmore Island. Neilus is my mom's younger brother and Mom and Annie have always been closer than sisters.

When I was three, Mom and Dad moved back to Ireland and they settled in Galway. Their prime incentive for moving home was to educate their family. They had their final child Kevin, in Galway, five years after me, whom we tortured with tales of rescue adoption until he was too old to believe us.

My parents bought Reilly's Hotel in 1976. They renamed it "The Holiday Hotel" because they had their first date in the Holiday Ballroom in Chicago. The nightclub that they added to the hotel, they called "Cheers" for the most part. The Holiday Hotel is situated in the heart of Salthill, two doors down from Seapoint, and it helped rear and educate all five of us.

My parents sold the hotel a few years ago and the house that my dad attached to it in which we all grew up, was recently demolished. Apartments are going up in its place in keeping with the new trend of the area.

Growing up in Ireland I had the best of both worlds because I spent the winters in Galway with Mom, Dad and my brothers, and the summers in Arranmore with Annie and Neilus.

I was educated in Galway by the Dominican nuns in Taylors Hill, and I really loved it. My brothers went to St. Joseph's or the "Bish" as it is known, and they turned out to be keen oarsmen. I played hockey, and I clearly remember racing home on my bike after training to beat the six o'clock bells of the Angelus.

I graduated from Taylors in 1989 and went to University College Galway (UCG). I had no idea what or who I wanted to be and had less interest in growing up. I studied Economics, Sociology and Politics. After completing my second year there I decided to go tulip picking in Holland for the summer. My brother Vince drove me to Tulla in County Clare to sign up, but I was too late because all of the places were taken. That meant that I would have to work in the Hotel for the entire summer of 1991 and I was not a bit happy about that.

Meanwhile, there was a very happy vagabond drifting around the South of Ireland. He was just about out of money, so he decided to stop and have a pint of Guinness in the Holiday Hotel. Mom was working the bar and they started to talk. His name was Noel Bradley.

Noel was on his fourth year break from his studies in Mechanical Engineering at Jordanstown, outside Belfast. He was originally from Belfast and he was raised in "the troubles." His parents owned a chain of shoe shops and were blown up a couple of times, so eventually they decided to get out. They moved to Fahan, on the Donegal side of the Derry border. Noel had recently returned to Ireland after a stint in London, and he was delighted to be back on Irish soil.

Salthill is a beautiful seaside resort on the west coast of Ireland. It is basically one long street off a promenade that looks out onto Galway Bay. The street contains many hotels, restaurants and arcades and behind that street, many residential areas are scattered. Noel explained to my mom that he had just asked most of the hotels on the street for work because he was low on cash and that he decided to stop for a rest before resuming his job hunt.

The Holiday Hotel is comparatively small. It is a ten bedroom hotel with a restaurant, two bars and a nightclub. Like many small family businesses, it was always too small to pay for enough staff to run itself, and give Mom and Dad an easy life. The summer months however attract many tourists to Salthill, which meant that extra staff needed to be hired.

As Mom listened to Noel that day in June 1991, she thought about his poor mother worrying about him and she instantly decided to do right by her. She fed Noel a home cooked meal and offered him a full time job in the bar, starting the following week. She also set him up with very reasonable accommodation and rent in her old house in Riverside.

Noel was a very happy man.

As with every year in the hotel it took time for the summer team of 1991 to form. It would have been a summer like all others, I am sure, only for my brother Vince was hired as night porter. I don't think that he was alone for one second of the night shift ever and I am certain that none of us slept very much for the entire summer.

My eldest brother Pat was stand-in Disc Jockey and although I tried to be miserable working there, they made it very difficult. I did make a few last ditch attempts to do something else with the summer but failed. Hence, I was late joining the team. For the evening shift, there were two bars, the quiet front and the disco back. For my first shift I landed the disco back with Noel.

The back bar looked out over a long rectangular dance floor that was surrounded with booths. The walls had mirrors for wallpaper to make the room look bigger. I hated polishing those mirrors. Anyway, I remember introducing myself to Noel. I was glad that the music was so loud because I was not in the mood for socializing.

The first thing I noticed about Noel was that he was obviously high on life. He was dancing. The disco back was the fun bar and we had fun working it. I also noticed with relief that Noel was a competent barman. Actually, he was a great barman. He knew how to make every cocktail to perfection and he was fast. He had all the signs of a natural and I was relieved that he didn't need training.

The music usually stopped at about 1:30 a.m. and we generally had the place cleaned up and ready for the breakfast crew by 3:00 a.m. That is when Vince would start the night porter shift. He made it difficult for anyone to go home by starting some crazy competition or insisting that we had something important to celebrate. So, we all hung out a lot that summer in the middle of the night keeping Vince company.

Vince and Noel became good friends early on. They initiated a joint quest for the perfect woman and they were most entertaining. They tried very hard to find the perfect woman and amazingly many women were willing to try out for the title, but, as the summer passed they still hadn't found what they were looking for. Then, the strangest thing happened.

It was our tradition by the end of July to jump into Galway Bay pre dawn. One early dawn we were swimming in the Bay and Noel kissed me. That was it. He declared to everyone the following evening that his quest for the perfect woman had ended. We just clicked. We really clicked. For the rest of the summer we took our days off together and we worked the same shifts. We became inseparable and I know that some people referred to us as "the painful couple."

Summer was coming quickly to an end and that meant reality for most. I had another year to complete in UCG. Late August, Noel asked me to marry him and I said yes. We needed a plan so we made one. Noel decided that he wanted to go back to Jordanstown to finish his degree so that he could get a better job. It would be the following year before he could do that, as he had to reapply. I told him that I would study with him in Jordanstown. I decided that I would study my Masters' degree there. Meanwhile, he could work the bars in Galway until I completed my BA in UCG. That was our plan. It all made perfect sense and we were so happy. I remember feeling so incredibly happy. I will never forget that feeling.

Then, Noel's left foot went to sleep and would not wake up.

Chapter 2

It was one of the very last days of August 1991 when Noel came to work earlier than usual and mentioned casually that his left foot felt like it was sleeping for the past couple of days. We all joked about it and told him to slap it around a bit. We told him that it was good that at least part of him was getting some rest. Nobody took it in any way serious.

Summer ended, the team split up, and everyone went their separate ways. I went back to UCG and Noel stayed on working for Mom and Dad in the hotel. He reapplied to Jordanstown to finish his degree as we had planned and he was instantly accepted. He was due to start his final year of Mechanical Engineering in September 1992 as a mature student. He was twenty-five and I was twenty-one.

In order for me to study in Jordanstown I needed a scholarship. To guarantee a scholarship I needed a 1st Class BA, so I worked for it and I got it. I phoned Jordanstown and a lady from their administration staff offered me a European scholarship on the spot. It covered all fees and it also included ninety-five pounds sterling a week spending money. That was enough money for both of us to live on if we in worked the student union bar a night or two a week. It was more than we could have hoped for and I was ecstatic. I instantly accepted her offer and she promised me that she would forward all of the documentation in writing so that I could formally sign for it.

The Masters offered by Jordanstown was exactly the course that I was looking for. I wanted to study Computing and Information Systems so I could actually do something at the end of it, like write a program, or at least turn on a computer. The job market needed such talents and were offering competitive salaries so I was excited.

I waited every day of summer 1992 for the written confirmation that was promised. It fast became late summer. A new team had formed and gelled in the hotel. Vince was no longer night porter and Pat was no longer DJ. I silently noticed that Noel was still slapping his foot around trying to wake it up. It was time to move on. But the letter never came.

The disaster that followed is one true testament in my mind to the fact that everything happens for a reason. I don't believe in coincidence. Early September came and I called Jordanstown to let them know that I never received any written confirmation. They assured me that they sent it to me but because I had not responded in time, they offered my scholarship to someone else. It was no longer available. I hung up the phone and I was very angry because I knew that something was not quite right.

I ransacked the mail and asked everyone if they had seen a letter from Belfast addressed to me during the summer. Nobody claimed to have seen it.

I went out to the reception area and Mom called me over to the fireplace to talk to me. She looked visibly shaken. Mom told me that she received the letter and burned it. She told me that she was sorry and explained that she panicked. She said that she didn't want me to go to Belfast when I had my choice of universities and scholarships. She explained that it had nothing to do with Noel, she was always very fond of him. She simply didn't want me anywhere near the bombings. I was very angry. I could not understand her actions and I lashed out untamed. Mom is tough but she cried. I knew that she was sorry but I could not stop venting.

Noel arrived to work later that evening and I told him what had happened. He didn't consider it a big deal because he understood my mother's concerns. Noel said that he would still finish his degree in Jordanstown and that I could study a Masters in Galway.

I had my heart set on the course in Jordanstown at this stage so I phoned the University again. I asked them if the same scholarship would be available to me the following year. They said that they would hold one for me considering the circumstances. I asked them to please do that and I decided to take a year out from my studies to travel.

To this day my mom has not forgiven herself for burning the letter, and it seemed to her at the time that my year out would never end. She deeply feared I would not return to my studies. If ever anything bad happens to me now, I always wonder how I will look at it after a few years of hindsight. Looking back now, Mom burning the letter, was the best thing that could possibly have happened to us in the long run. It was that year out that led to a particular chain of events that could never have occurred otherwise.

September 1992 came and Noel started his final year of Engineering at Jordanstown. I planned on touring France, but instead I ended up drifting around Ireland for the year working odd jobs here and there.

By the end of his course, Noel's left leg was sleeping from the knee down. Looking back, you would think that he or I would have addressed the issue by this point. We just didn't.

Noel got a job in Belfast with a small company shortly after he graduated, and I started my Masters' degree in Computing and Information Systems in September 1993 as our new plan dictated. I remember noticing towards the end of my studies that Noel's balance was very bad after a couple of drinks. Still, I did not address it because I could not address it.

I went to the summer Job Fare in Jordanstown on June 12th 1993, and I was offered a job in London with a financial software company called Wilco. It was the only year that they ever interviewed in Belfast. Had I completed the course a year earlier I would never have heard of Wilco and to make a long story short I would never have landed in New York and I would never have met Dr. Bihari. If I moved to the States independently, without Wilco, it would have been Chicago that I would have targeted because I have a lot of family based there still. Anyway, Wilco offered me a job on the spot and it was just the job I was looking for, but I was not too keen on the idea of moving to London at the time. However, the company Noel was working for went bankrupt and he was out of work and finding it difficult to get another job so money was tight.

We needed a new plan, so we made one. Noel decided that he wanted to do a Masters' degree so that he could get a job. He landed a grant for the course I just completed and our new plan formed. I would accept the job in London. Noel would complete his Masters and then he would apply to Wilco for work the following year and join me in London.

We did not address his sleepy leg. I could not address it.

Chapter 3

I moved to London in September 1994 and Noel started his Masters' degree in Jordanstown. I was very lucky because my brother Pat was already set up in London. He was working for Dorling Kindersley and living in Clapham Common. He took me under his wing. I loved living with Pat. There are many sides to Pat and he is always interesting and fun to be with. I flew to Belfast regularly to see Noel and we were constantly on the phone to each other.

Early 1995, Noel called me. His left foot was completely numb at this stage and his right foot was starting to go to sleep. He made an appointment at the Royal Hospital in Belfast because it was time to address the issue. The outcome of his appointment still puzzles me.

They did an MRI and told Noel that they didn't think that he had Multiple Sclerosis (MS) but they could not be sure. They said that they look at three things to diagnose MS, namely a clinical evaluation, an MRI and a lumbar puncture to examine the fluid in the spine. If you show signs of MS in any two of these then you have MS.

Years later we showed his MRI from the Royal, to a neurologist in London who could clearly see scarring, indicating that the MRI showed signs of MS. I am surprised that the clinical evaluation in Belfast did not concur and also surprised that they did not do a lumbar puncture. However, it was 1995 and pre all MS medications. There was no treatment, so there was no rush to diagnose because there was nothing to offer.

The doctor left Noel in limbo by saying that there was a good chance that the numbness would go away but pointed out that it may get worse and if that started to happen, then they would look into it further. So, they basically told Noel to carry on with everything as normal and to hope for the best. I am an expert at hoping for the best so I was completely elated with the news. Everything was going to be just fine in my mind.

Summer 1995 came and Noel opted to complete his dissertation in Thessalonica, Greece. I took two weeks off and joined him there. It was very hot. I clearly remember noticing that if there was a stool available he would always use it.

I did not address it because I could not address it. Everything was going to be just fine.

Noel completed his Masters with distinction and Wilco offered him a job as we had hoped. He moved to London and started working for Wilco in October 1995. In January 1996 he bought me an engagement ring and we planned our wedding for October 1996. I knew that something was not right but for the life of me I could not put my finger on it. I developed severe panic attacks that summer and had to take off work. I jumped on a plane and went home to Galway.

It felt great to be home. There is no place like home. Mom and Dad were so happy so see me and could not do enough. My brother Phil was studying medicine at the time and it became his turn to take me under his wing. He was working at his desk in his room that he used to share with Pat. It had two twin beds overlooking the promenade. I loved that view of Galway Bay. I entered and stretched out on Pat's bed and told Phil that I was losing my mind. He was surprised but happy to see me and asked me to tell him everything. I was as honest as I could be at the time.

I told him that it all started on the tube ride to work one morning. The underground tubes in London during rush hour are packed tight and nobody speaks to anybody. I said that I was standing near the exit holding on to a ceiling handrail when I felt the whole world spin. My heart thumped so loud that it echoed in my head. My breathing became fast and uncontrolled and I broke into an instant sweat. I told Phil that I thought that I was going to faint. The gut wrenching furnace of fear I felt inside that made me want to sprint for miles was the only thing that prevented me from keeling over. It was absolutely terrifying.

As time passed these episodes became more frequent so I went to a doctor in Sydenham, London, who referred me to a psychiatrist at the hospital. I was annoyed that he thought the problem was all in my mind but I decided to see the psychiatrist to prove him wrong. I never did see the psychiatrist. I went for my appointment but could not wait in the waiting room because there were too many crazies there. There was a guy screaming at a wall, another banging his head off a chair and a lady having a full scale conversation with herself, she even moved position to answer herself. They were all products of lonely London, all people whom the system had failed. They epitomized everything I hated about London and how it operates. I left.

I called Noel and told him that I was going to the airport. I had to get out of London. I had to go home. I also called my manager in Wilco on my way to the airport. She was wonderful. She told me not to worry about work and to take as long as I needed.

Phil looked at me and told me that I would be fine. I was shocked at how calm he was. I was also shocked by the speed of his diagnosis. Then I realized that he related far too well to my situation. He told me that I was having panic attacks. He shared with me that my maternal grandmother lived with them most of her life and that he was also prone to them. We shared the annoying panic attack gene.

I was wired at this stage. I had not slept in days because every time I was about to drift off my heart would start to race and a gripping fear would make me pace the room. I couldn't eat because every time I tried, my stomach would clench with the same invisible fear. I was glad to lose a few pounds before the wedding but I was very aware that I was losing my strength. Phil gave me valium to knock me out but initially I didn't want to take it. I wanted to beat the attacks on my own now that I knew that it was a mental issue. I asked Phil if he popped valium nightly and he said that he didn't, but he told me that Grandma did. I asked him how he conquered his anxiety and he told me that he prayed. I did not understand what he was talking about. I popped a couple of valium and went to my childhood room and slept like a baby. The next morning at breakfast Phil started to ask me about Noel.

I talked and talked about Noel. I talked about how well he was doing at work. He was climbing the ladder fast. He was proving to be a computer whiz and he loved his job. I talked about our nights out in the West End and all the friends we made. I talked about how he went out one morning to buy me an engagement ring like he was going out to buy a loaf of bread. I joked that I should never have accepted the ring until he got down on one knee. Getting down on one knee is just not Noel's style. I talked about everything, but I did not talk about the numbness in his legs. I could not talk about it. I didn't even know that I could not talk about it.

Phil pressed me a bit. He specifically asked if Noel's foot ever woke up. I told him that it didn't, but I immediately clarified that it was nothing because he got checked out at the Royal in Belfast and they told him to carry on as normal.

"Thank God it was nothing!" I said.

Phil pressed more. I told him that the numbness had spread a little but assured him that it was nothing. Then, Phil asked me if Noel had health and life insurance. I laughed and said no. Phil said that it would be a good idea for Noel to get all of his insurance papers in order before going for any more tests because it seemed clear to him that Noel had Multiple Sclerosis.

I cracked up laughing.

I asked Phil if he had read the "good bedside manner" chapter of the "How to Be a Doctor" book , and if so he should brush up on it. Phil can be serious. Phil was deadly serious. I told him that he was crazy but assured him that I appreciated his concern. This time he was just so far off the mark. Noel was fine. The neurologist said so. Everything was going to be just fine. I just had to find a way to switch off the panic attack gene and get on with my life. I had a party to go to in October. I was getting married.

Noel phoned me every evening after work and that night in late June 1996 I told him that poor Phil thought that Noel had MS. Noel was calm. He said that if he had MS then he had MS, to him it was not a big deal. He told me that everyone has to play the hand they are dealt in life. Then, he asked me if I had sorted my head out.

"No!" I laughed, but then I told him that I was going to head up to Arranmore and get to the bottom of it. I explained that I was going to ask Grandma for the cure. Until then I would get by on valium.

Chapter 4

I love Arranmore. Annie and Neilus own the island restaurant and it is always my first stop when I get off the ferry boat. Attached to the restaurant there is a video games room with a candy counter, and even now all of the island children gather and play there just as I did with my peers growing up. I laugh every time I visit because I usually get caught at that candy counter. Every family operates differently. I have many memories of falling for the "stand there for five minutes" routine, both in the bar in Galway and the restaurant in Arranmore. After five hours of standing I can still hear my dad laughing and asking me, "did you learn anything?"

I arrived in Arranmore and dropped my bags in Annie's restaurant. I avoided the candy counter and I headed up the bray to Grandma's house on the bridge. Grandma was 95. She was always very strong and insisted that she was never overweight, she was just big boned with fluid retention. A bird could eat more than her she claimed. She looked weaker than usual and told me that she was ready to die. I asked her to hang on until the party in October but she teased that she had her fill of weddings and funerals.

I asked her if she ever had panic attacks. She asked me what they were, so I explained, and she understood. She told me that I was blocking something and that I had to figure out the puzzle for myself. She said that it may take years and that indeed I may never get to the bottom of it. Then, I asked her if she took valium. She said that she didn't know the names of all of the pills that she took. She knew exactly the size, color, shape and purpose of each one, just not the names. Nobody could ever give her a placebo. I looked at her supply and told her that she did take valium.

"Mary dear, that has been my sleeping pill of many years," she said.

I told her that I didn't want to be on pills for a mental issue and she laughed so heartily. I asked her what she thought I could be blocking and she told me that she hadn't a clue.

"Maybe you have a bad dose of the wedding jitters," she said.

We laughed a lot together. That evening we just hung out and drank hot chocolate. Sadly, that was our last visit together. Grandma died in July that year.

I headed back to Galway and asked Phil to explain to me how to deal with the attacks. He gave me a two week supply of valium and told me to pray. I told him that I didn't want to pray.

"Then you better pray to want to pray," he replied. It was time to go back to London.

Noel met me at Heathrow airport. It was obvious at this stage that standing for long periods of time was starting to get very difficult for him. I made a silent mental note. We were so happy to see each other. I was looking forward to going back to work and our wedding was approaching. I had a wedding to organize and Noel had a honeymoon to book. Everything was going to be just fine.

I eased back into work and started to master the panic attacks when the valium ran out. It was difficult to say the least. I did have to pray.

October came so we flew to Galway. We had a wonderful wedding. Vince was Noel's best man and he gave a comical speech with much reference to their antics when they worked in the hotel together. Everybody had a good time. It was the first Boyle wedding.

I distinctly remember the wedding dance with Noel because he stood on my feet three or four times. I had a mild panic attack after the dance but nobody even noticed because I had a coping mechanism in place at that point. I had mastered them. I used to focus on a short private prayer and they would pass.

I always laugh when I remember our wedding day because towards the end, my brother Pat joined the band and made everyone forget about the video and go completely crazy. It is the funniest wedding video I think I have ever seen. It is the video that taught us all how not to dance at weddings.

After a wonderful honeymoon in Jamaica, Noel and I returned to London and went back to work. A year passed and by then Noel was completely numb from both knees down. We took the Eurostar train to Paris from London for a weekend for our first anniversary, and I remember he had great trouble with the steps of the Eiffel Tower. I also remember that he found it difficult to stand for a few hours when we were out and if a stool was available he automatically sat.

On occasion he would test himself by running across the park in London. Noel never talked about it, and I never asked. I simply could not ask. It was completely invisible to everyone and very easy to forget about. The panic attacks were a rarity but they still lingered.

Christmas 1997 came and we found out that I was pregnant. Noel was absolutely over the moon. We both were. We were ecstatic. I had a very healthy pregnancy and I insisted that Noel attended the birth. I figured that it couldn't be that bad an experience. I actually thought that he may even enjoy it.

I finally went into labor September 2nd 1998 and I paged Noel. His mother Maura was visiting us at the time and we always laugh at how I kicked off the labor. I basically walked a marathon until it started. As soon as I was admitted, Noel arrived at Kings Hospital in London. He had developed foot drop of the left leg but it was so slight that nobody would ever even notice it and it was only ever apparent when he was under great stress or over tired. But it was there.

The labor lasted sixteen hours and the epidural failed. The cord got caught around the neck of the baby and her heartbeat kept dipping very low. Things were tense for a while. At last, Annie Kate arrived but she was completely blue and she didn't cry, so they took her away to a corner of the room to work on her. Noel very nearly fainted, he went pale and started to sweat. Thank God, Annie Kate turned a healthy pink and started to roar. When Noel's color returned, I remember thinking that he looked like the happiest dad on the planet.

He was so proud of his daughter. Annie Kate was purposely named after my Aunt Annie and her mother Kate.

Shortly after Annie Kate was born a close childhood friend of mine, Coirle, visited us in London. She told me that her sister married a wonderful guy named Robert. She shared with me how much in love Robert and her sister were, but also that she was concerned for them both because Robert was diagnosed with Multiple Sclerosis. She described his symptoms as having numb feet. She said that he was wobbly after a couple of drinks and very tired in the evenings. I asked her what exactly MS was. She told me that she didn't really know, but just knew that as MS went, Robert was very lucky. She said that as MS went Robert had the best possible type. I really felt bad for Coirle's sister and Robert on hearing the news.

"That is a very tough hand," I said.

I told Coirle that it made me appreciate having a healthy husband and child all the more.

"Good health is everything!" I stated, and Coirle completely agreed.

At this stage, Noel and I were living in a beautiful company apartment in Surrey Quays in London. We were waiting on a transfer to Dublin. Wilco had plans to open an office in Dublin and I was very happy about that. I desperately wanted to raise my family in Ireland. I really wanted to be near Mom, Dad, Annie and Neilus, and I felt that I had traveled enough. Things could not have been better. Then came November 1998.

Mom and Annie came to visit us briefly in London to meet Annie Kate. We had a lot of fun together as always. Shortly after that visit, Noel had to go on a business trip to Frankfurt and by the time he returned his symptoms were very pronounced and very visible. The culprit of the panic attacks was about to come out into the open and that is when the real roller coaster took off.

Chapter 5

Noel came home to our apartment in Surrey Quays after work one day in November 1998 with a staggering gait. He looked like he was about to fall over on every step. He used the walls of the apartment when he was in the hall to get around because the numbness was spreading rapidly up his legs. It was very scary to watch.

He staggered into the living room and started playing with Annie Kate. Amazingly, he joked and laughed with her as if he didn't have a care in the world. Equally amazingly, I didn't say a thing. I just went into the kitchen and started to cook the dinner as usual. Then, as I peeled the potatoes and focused on that short prayer, Noel called into the kitchen from the living room. He said that maybe I should make an appointment with a doctor for him. I agreed and continued to prepare our meal and he continued to play with our baby.

I never did take Phil's advice regarding insurance so we didn't have private health insurance which meant that we were reliant on the National Health Service (NHS) in London. We went to a doctor in Surrey Quays and he told us that Noel had to see a neurologist. The waiting list to see a neurologist on the NHS at the time was about eight months. That was too long for us to wait so we decided to go private and pay in full. We met with one of the top neurologists in London. He reviewed the MRI from the Royal in Belfast, performed a series of cognitive tests, did a lumbar puncture and took a very detailed health history.

I will never forget going in for the results. We entered his office and he asked us to sit down. Noel was holding Annie Kate. The neurologist looked happy and said that he was incredibly relieved because he was convinced that Noel had a brain tumor initially. He said that there was no brain tumor and qualified his excitement with that fact that Noel had Multiple Sclerosis. I broke down. I had a complete meltdown. Noel was calm.

"Shit happens," he said.

That is all he said.

I calmed down, realizing immediately that I needed to know absolutely everything. The neurologist said that Noel had primary progressive MS and that he would just keep getting worse and worse over time. He said that he could not give us a timeline of progression and explained that with MS each person is different. He wasn't certain if Noel's MS would progress slowly or quickly but he was certain that Noel's MS would progress.

Noel asked if Annie Kate was at risk of contracting MS and the neurologist assured him that as far as he knew, she was safe, but added that Noel's siblings had a higher risk than normal of developing MS. I asked the neurologist what we could do to fix it. I asked what medication was available. He replied that there was nothing we could do to fix it and that there were no medications to help his diagnosis.

On hearing that I really lost control. "How could there be nothing?" I yelled.

The neurologist said that if Noel had the relapsing remitting form of MS, there were various beta interferon medications, but for Noel there was nothing because he had chronic MS. I felt that the diagnosis was worse than a brain tumor at the beginning because there was no operation to even try to fix it all.

Noel thanked the neurologist and we left. I was a mess. I was a complete mess. Noel told me to cheer up.

"It could be worse," Noel said.

"How so?" I asked. "What on earth could be worse?"

"You could have it," he said.

"But why do you have it?" I said. "Why you?"

'"Why not me?" he replied.

That night, after Noel put Annie Kate to sleep he stumbled into the living room and found me crying. I found his diagnosis so difficult to accept. I asked him how on earth could he be so calm about it all. I really wondered what was going on in his mind. He sat down and told me that he would share his secret. He told me that nothing could bring him down ever again and he would tell me why. I knew his life history but never knew his real perception of it all.

Noel told me that when he was growing up in Belfast, the lack of respect for human life always deeply saddened him. He had a pretty lonely childhood. Then, when he went to boarding school in Newry, there was an alcoholic priest, Fr Finnegan, who inappropriately fondled many of the young boys in his trust. Noel was one of his victims. That experience set Noel on a course of self destruction. When Noel entered Jordanstown the first time, he was spiraling downhill. He left his studies and tried to escape in London. There, he worked some building sites and many bars and he became deeply depressed. He tried to end his life by jumping off a building. He hit rock bottom. He still questions if that fall triggered his MS. Anyway, shortly after surviving that experience he figured everything out. I suppose you could say that he had an epiphany.

He woke up one morning and saw God in everything. Every living thing suddenly mattered to him. He came to see himself as just a small part of a wonderful creation and he became very grateful for every breath. He developed a huge appreciation for life. He suddenly saw the beauty in everyone, every single person, and gained a new respect for the gift of life. He forgave Fr Finnegan. He came to believe that the priest was lost and deserved help.

That night, Noel told me that no matter what he is thrown in life, it didn't matter in the grand scheme of things. He was determined to live right, as if he had a test to pass. If he had one day, two or ten left to live, he was determined to make the most of every second and to keep going and going until he could not go any more. It was that simple. He said that he could deal with having MS because he was alive. He said that in his mind he had suffered worse. He told me that he had never in his life been happier than then because he had a wife and a child whom he loved deeply and that was all that mattered. He thought himself so much luckier than most.

"MS is not a big deal," he stated.

That day marked the last of all of my panic attacks. They were firmly put to rest.

Chapter 6

I was really looking forward to our transfer to Dublin. We would have a great deal of family support in Ireland. Then something happened in the stock market in Tokyo late 1998 and the effect rippled across all of the stock markets. A Wilco office in Dublin was no longer a viable option and that meant that there was to be no transfer home.

It was coming up to Christmas 1998 and my brother Vince was getting married so we decided to fly home for the wedding. Just before we left, Noel was offered a job transfer to New York. Wilco wanted him to start January 1999. We decided to discuss it over the holidays so we flew home. I was very tired and Noel's gait was very unbalanced to say the least, but we were very happy. We truly were happy, we were a family.

We arrived home and as always it was great to be home. Vince was delighted to have found his perfect woman. I set them up some years ago. Helen studied with me at UCG and I knew that she would be the perfect woman for Vince. Vince is a really wonderful guy. My four brothers are just great guys and I don't think that I am being biased in saying that because anybody who knows them would agree. I think that they are brilliant in everything they do.

The wedding party all gathered in Galway and the celebrations started. Everybody was so obviously and naturally taken back by the decline in Noel. They didn't know what to do or say, so everybody more or less ignored it. We all carried on as normal. We sat in the living room with the large windows looking over Galway Bay and told funny stories. Annie Kate was the star attraction, everybody instantly just loved her.

Later that night, I headed out for a bit to catch up with an old friend, who was just back from the States. She was home for the christening of her first child. I called out to her house and her sister was there. Her sister was a physiotherapist in London and I told her about Noel. She told me that in her experience and knowledge Noel had five more years left to live. She told me that nobody ever tells patients with chronic MS the truth, but assured me that within five years he would be bedridden with feeding tubes. I couldn't take it in. I left.

Thank God Annie and Neilus were staying with Mom and Dad for the wedding. I arrived home and signaled Mom and Annie from the living room. I told them what I heard and I broke down again. Annie told me that she knew people with MS who lived to be a ripe old age. Mom told me that she was going to visit the Poor Clare Nuns in the morning and that everything would be just fine.

"God never gives you more than you can handle," she said.

I told Mom and Annie that I was not going to make Vince's wedding because I couldn't. I didn't want to wreck it on them. Equally, I did not want Noel to realize my true messed up mental state. I desperately wanted to be strong and happy for him so I instructed them that it was their job to cover for me by whatever means necessary. I needed time, so I went to bed early with Annie Kate and an apparent headache. It felt good to have Mom and Annie support me and I slept well.

The next day Mom went to visit the Poor Clares. The Poor Clares are a community of nuns that have been in Galway since 1642. Their vowed life of poverty, chastity and obedience is lived in enclosure. It is common practice in Galway to ask these women to pray for special intentions. Their monastery is based in Nuns Island. The Poor Clares gave Mom the name of a doctor in Cork, Dr. Muriel. They told Mom that Dr. Muriel has chronic MS and she had asked them to give her number out to anyone in need of MS counseling. Mom, Annie and I went to the reception of the hotel for privacy and I dialed the number.

I thought that it was going to be a difficult phone call. I felt dreadful that this woman had this disease and had no idea how to ask her how long she had left to live, much less her present quality of life. I had no idea when the number was handed into the Poor Clares and in my mind I honestly questioned if she was still alive.

Thankfully, Dr. Muriel answered the phone. I introduced myself and told her that my husband was just diagnosed with chronic MS. I explained that my mom got her number from the Poor Clares in Galway, and then I asked her if she was willing to share her story. She was wonderful. She gave me all the strength I needed to go to Vince and Helen's wedding. She told me that she had chronic MS for twenty-five years and that she was still self-sufficient. She said that she had to give up her medical practice but assured me that she really enjoyed life despite a walker and wheelchair. She told me not to give up. She gave me hope. When I hung up, Mom, Annie and I were so relieved. Dr. Muriel was a Godsend.

The next day, December 28th 1998, Vince and Helen got married. It was a beautiful wedding and everyone enjoyed it. Helen knows how to do things just right and we all knew how to behave for the video.

Afterwards, Noel and I told everyone that we were going to move to New York. Noel was so set on the idea that I didn't have the heart to stop him. I dreaded it. Yet, in my mind he only had a few more years of quality living left, so I figured that he might as well travel the world when he still could. I decided that I didn't have a great need to settle until Annie Kate started school and that was a long time off. Also, the company had only offered Noel a one year contract so I thought that I would be back in Ireland before I knew it. Furthermore, I was still on maternity leave and I did not want to leave Annie Kate for a second. I did not want to go back to work and the salary increase Noel was promised upon his transfer would make it easier for me to stay at home. I tried to look at the transfer as an adventure filled with stories that I could share.

My family was tactfully deeply concerned. Vince begged me in private not to go. He desperately wanted to help us out. He wanted to be there for us. He wanted us near him. Vince is the worrier of the family and the last to be told anything. He was the child that hung out on the windowsill of Mom and Dad's bedroom if ever they went out for an evening, which was a rarity. I remember he used to run into my room to wake me to tell me that everything was okay when they arrived home safely.

Noel's family also came to Galway that Christmas and they could not believe that we were thinking of moving to New York, but like the rest they put on a brave face and wished us the best.

Early January 1999, we flew back to London and started to prepare for the transfer to New York. Noel's legs were completely numb but still strong at this stage. His plan was to work on walking again with the new lack of sensation over the next few months.

Chapter 7

That January, Noel flew to New York a week ahead of Annie Kate and me, to sort out our accommodation. A U.S. Company, Automatic Data Processing (ADP) bought Wilco a few years earlier. That meant that all of the benefits for ADP employees were made available to Wilco employees automatically, without exception or medical test, on transferring to the U.S.. Noel was offered all ADP company benefits so he maxed out on health and life insurance.

We settled into a company apartment on Monroe Street in Hoboken. It was about ten blocks from the Path train that Noel needed to use to get to work. It snowed a lot that January and he fell quite a few times walking that distance. To be honest, I have no idea how he walked that far in the snow at the time without breaking his neck. I bought him an umbrella that could double as a cane but he wouldn't use it.

I had visited Hoboken years before through work and I loved it. It is a trendy place with cozy bars and restaurants and very convenient for people who work in New York City. This time I didn't like it. In my mind it was not baby friendly and our second floor apartment in a building with no elevator had windows that wouldn't open. I hated that. It was quite a workout coming and going from the apartment with all of the baby gear. I also hated that. Annie Kate had the best stroller, but the weight of it was never taken into consideration on purchase. Also, we didn't have a car. Again I hated that. But what I hated most of all was watching Noel drag himself up the stairs in the evening after work.

Despite all of that we were happy. We honestly were. I was very tired but happy overall. Noel was unsteady but he never complained about it. He was still high on life. I admit that there were times that I broke down on my own and cried, but I vowed that he would never see me cry. I was determined to be strong for Noel and I knew that I was getting stronger day by day. I could feel it. I really started to toughen up.

About two weeks after we had settled into Hoboken I found out why I was so tired. I was pregnant again. Noel was once again over the moon. I was delighted also as I wanted Annie Kate to have a close sibling. I didn't want her to be an only child. My pregnancy confirmed my decision that it was time to find a better place to live and make the most of the year. There was no way I was going to bring a second baby home to that apartment.

I didn't know anybody in Hoboken. I didn't want to know anybody. One morning, I headed to the train station with Annie Kate after Noel went to work and I bought a map. I then took a train timetable and went home to study it and I came up with a plan. Every morning I would go to the station after Noel went to work and I would hit each town, one by one, on the Bergen Line until I found one I liked. I had to keep in mind that Noel had to commute this distance on top of his current commute so I was hoping to find a town nearby that was baby friendly and had a furnished house to rent beside the station with windows that opened. So, every morning Annie Kate and I searched. It took a while.

Then, one cold, clear morning the train stopped at Ridgewood, New Jersey. I didn't only like it, I loved it. It was beautiful and really clean. It was spacious yet quaint. It was perfect.

We moved to Ridgewood in February 1999 and settled into 237 Godwin Avenue. It was a three family home and we rented the upstairs section. The house was very near the station and every window opened. I thought that Ridgewood was very baby friendly and I felt a new lease of life. Noel walked to and from the station every morning and evening. Although he never regained any sensation back in his legs, he succeeded in teaching himself to walk again.

I was determined for Noel to visit another neurologist. To find the best one I decided that I needed a car. To get a car I needed a U.S. license, and to get a U.S. license, I needed to convert my London license, and to convert my London license, I needed to do a written test. Shortly after we moved to Ridgewood, we met the elderly couple living in the downstairs section of 237 Godwin. They were Marge and Joe from a neighboring town. Their house had burnt down and it was in the process of being rebuilt. Marge and I became instant friends. She is a retired school teacher. She didn't have an easy life by any means. She had two sons, and one died when he was twenty-six. He was the picture of health but choked on a piece of meat and died. It was such a sudden tragedy that most people would never overcome, but Marge did. Also, her husband Joe was battling with Rheumatoid Arthritis and in bad shape. Despite all of that, Marge was very happy. She oozed a gentle inner peace that I loved.

Marge took me under her wing and showed me all the ropes. I got my license with Annie Kate on my knee for the written test and I bought a car, a 1991 Buick Century. I remember buying the car. It was from the Buick dealer near the train station in Ridgewood, on Broad Street. The salesman asked me to take it for a test drive but I told him that there was no need for a test drive as it looked fine. I had never driven an automatic before and I was afraid that I would crash it. I paid him five grand in cash and he gave me the keys.

It was a nervous ride home and Annie Kate screamed in the back the whole way. But at last we had a car. Marge laughed at the story of purchase and then taught me how to drive on the highways. Noel could not drive the Buick. He could not feel the peddles properly with his feet.

As soon as I had transport, I started to investigate neurologists. I firmly believed that if anywhere could treat Noel, it was America.

I started with the phone book because I didn't have access to a computer. I was not familiar with the area so I simply called every neurologist in the book to see if they accepted our insurance and asked what the wait time for an appointment was. When I had narrowed the selection, I drove by certain offices and ran in to get literature from their office to get a feel of their qualifications, history, specialties and patient numbers. None of them had much information, to be honest. Some told me about the standard medications for MS but it became clear that America did not know of a cure.

I finally settled for a local group of neurologists. I called and I made an appointment for Noel for July 8th 1999. When I told Noel, he insisted that he did not want to go for the appointment. He tried to explain that he did not want to make MS his life. He figured that the neurologist in London knew his stuff and that we just had to accept it. It seemed completely futile to him he told me, to keep asking every doctor the same questions until I found one that would tell me what I wanted to hear. I told him that I just wanted a second opinion. I wanted to fight. He didn't.

I persisted and Noel finally gave in to humor me. He told me that I made his quest for an easy life very difficult. He eventually agreed that it was probably a good idea to have a neurologist in the States, so we went for the appointment.

I really liked Noel's new neurologist. He was very professional. He explained his impressive credentials and told us about all the meetings he attended with the MS experts of the world that kept him up to date with all the latest on MS research. He was the MS expert and I felt safe. He told Noel to start on Avonex, a weekly injection. It would most certainly slow the progression of his MS we were told. I felt so good leaving his office. At last we were doing something to fight back. Noel was calm and willing to give the shots a try.

July 1999 Noel started Avonex therapy. Avonex shots are intra muscular so the needle is about an inch long. They are referred to as beta interferon shots. That means that they suppress the immune system because it is widely believed that MS is the result of an overactive immune system. Clinical studies show that Avonex reduces the relapse rate in 35% of patients with MS. They do not stop the progression of MS or claim to. They slow it down for the lucky ones. I am sure that the neurologist explained all of that, but all I heard was that Avonex slows the progression of MS. I found out much later that Biogen, the makers of Avonex, state that it only works on relapsing remitting MS. It is not recommended for primary progressive MS but it was the neurologist's belief (which I appreciated so much at the time) that it was much better to do something instead of nothing. I had no idea what the actual odds of it working were. I knew nothing about the drug other than it was going to work. To keep me optimistic Biogen sent monthly newsletters filled with happy people with MS on Avonex.

I offered to administer Noel's shots and he accepted. We picked Saturday night because we were told that he would suffer flu like symptoms for a day or so after the needle, for up to nine months. I remember the first shot. Noel mixed it while Annie Kate was kicking on the floor in the living room in Godwin Avenue. My bump was also kicking and I read the pamphlet about ten times. It sounded simple. I just had to stick it in his thigh muscle. He handed me the needle and I stuck it in, released the shot and pulled it out. I pressed gently on the injection sight with a cloth that came as part of the kit, and there was very little blood. It seemed easy enough, but I was very relieved to get it over with. That time he didn't feel it.

Every Saturday, we alternated between his thighs although we could have used other muscles. There were times when I hit a vein and his blood spat everywhere and other times I hit a nerve or something and he'd jump his own height. It was always a relief to get the shot over with, but as time went on it just became part of our routine. I remember one beautiful Saturday morning we went to the Jersey shore, Point Pleasant. We stayed at the beach all day and then tried to book in somewhere for the night. The only available room was in a sleazy motel with a red flashing neon light. Annie Kate fell asleep so Noel measured the shot using the neon light. I remember thinking it very funny. When Annie Kate started to talk, she was fascinated with the procedure, so we put her in charge of the band-aid.

Initially, the flu like symptoms were very severe. Noel was feverish every Sunday for about a year but it didn't bother his spirits. He handled it very well. Tylenol and Advil pain relievers became a necessity, and as time went on he needed them less and less. The mental relief because we were actually doing something was huge to me. Our lives were busy so we didn't think about MS too much. Although busy, we were about to get even busier.

Chapter 8

September 25th 1999, I gave birth to Aisling. I didn't want Noel to attend the birth because I had learned that stress was not a good thing for MS. He also needed to stay home to look after Annie Kate. Mom, Dad, Annie and Neilus were visiting at the time, so Mom and Annie went to the hospital with me.

When Aisling was born, Annie Kate had just turned one, but she didn't walk until she was fourteen months. So, when the gang went back to Ireland and Noel returned to work I had very little time to obsess about his MS and life took over. I also felt that we were doing all that we could to combat his MS so I was more relaxed about it all and I trusted Noel's neurologist completely. I loved my girls and I was very happy. Once again things were very good and they were about to get a great deal better.

Marge and I spent many hours together debating life. One day when we were sorting out the problems of the world she told me that I should join the Mom's Group at Nativity Church in Midland Park. I told her that if ever we were organized enough on a Sunday morning we attended mass at Mount Carmel in Ridgewood. That was a rarity, but I knew a couple of people at this point and I didn't feel the need to branch out. Aisling was christened in Mount Carmel. Marge told me that I would really love Nativity. She explained that it was a smaller community with many stay at home moms.

"Every stay at home mom needs girlfriends," she said, "Nativity is not fancy, Mary, it is very simple."

I didn't feel that I needed anyone because I was very content hanging out with my girls and they kept me busy. However, I am sure that it was Marge who left the Nativity bulletin in my mailbox one morning late November 1999. I read it and saw that the Mom's

Group met on Wednesday mornings at 9:30 a.m. at the church with their children and drank coffee. I decided to take Marge's advice and check it out.

I always laugh when I remember this. I arrived at Nativity with a diaper bag around my neck, Annie Kate in one arm and Aisling in her car seat in my other arm. That was my normality. The room where the moms gathered was upstairs so I had to climb a flight of stairs and I was breathless by the time I got to the door. I walked in. It was a huge, plain, rectangular room. The smell of crayons, plastic and old books reminded me of my school in Ireland. There was a group of women sitting around laughing and many were holding young babies. It was noisy because boisterous toddlers were running around playing happily. One of the women came over to me and introduced herself briefly as Tia. She was in the middle of telling a funny story to the group, so as she was saying "hi" she was also turning her head back to the gang to finish her story. As if she knew me all of my life she took my children and told me to sit down.

I sat and she gave me a coffee and told me to relax for a couple of hours. I couldn't believe it. It was the best morning I'd had in years. I felt completely at home and I loved all of the women instantly. We bonded like teenagers and as time went on we often reverted to behaving as such. Rain, hail or shine I never missed Wednesday mornings at Nativity for the next while. Of course, I had no idea at the time how much I would rely on the women from Nativity in the future.

Noel's job was going very well at the time. One day in early December, he came home late and told me that ADP wanted him to stay in America for longer. Noel explained that he loved America. He also understood my desire to live in Ireland, so he decided that I should make the decision as to whether or not we should stay. I told him that I liked America too. I didn't want to move back to London with Wilco, and I figured that if we moved back to Ireland I would have to go back to work because he would not get the salary in Ireland to support us. I didn't want to put the girls in daycare when I had the option to stay at home with them. I also figured that even if Noel did get a salary in Ireland to support us. I would never have a network of stay at home moms like the group from Nativity because most young mothers in Ireland have to work now to raise their family. Another bonus about the States was that I felt that Noel was getting the best medical care there was. It made no sense in my mind to rock the boat.

I told him that I wanted to stay. Our lease in Ridgewood was due to expire in February 2000, so we decided to go house hunting.

At this stage, Noel's MS was very visible to everybody in the evenings and it was still progressing. His MS progression always just crept up on us. It was so slow that I used to only notice a decline when organizing my photo album. Then, he began to find the forty minute train journey home difficult if he didn't get a seat. I started picking him up at the station with the girls to make it easier for him because his legs started to get very tired and heavy at the end of the day. I could instantly tell by his gait when he came off the train whether or not he had a seat for the journey. I told him that he should get a cane so that people would know that he needed help, but he refused.

At times, when his walk became very bad, he would visit his neurologist and his neurologist would give him steroids. Noel loved steroids. They made him feel great. But, their effect was always short lived. Still, we were very busy and very happy and about to buy our first house. We didn't have time to dwell on his MS.

I went to playgroup one Wednesday as usual and mentioned to the Mom's Group that we were looking to buy a house. One of the mothers was a realtor and told me that a house near her was on the market. She said that her best friend had grown up in it and that it was reasonably priced. Noel and I went to check it out and we instantly put down a deposit. We moved onto Millington Drive on March 1st 2000, and we immediately started to add a dormer with the help of the realtor's husband.

For the longest time, our only piece of furniture was a three piece sectional. It was in our living room and consisted of a pull-out bed that we used nightly, and two recliners with a small table. Also in the living room, we set up a crib for Aisling, and in the back room, we set one up for Annie Kate. Our dormer expanded the two upstairs bedrooms and added a bathroom between them. Therefore, the upstairs had to be sealed off, and the workmen arrived every morning at 8:00 a.m. sharp for seven weeks and started hammering. The girls slept through some serious banging in the afternoons and if they couldn't sleep we all hung out at Tia's house.

I had to wake the girls up every morning to drive Noel to the station for 7:30 a.m.. We also picked him up every evening at 7:00 p.m..

One morning in spring, as we were heading to the car I felt really nauseous. Noel and I looked at each other and laughed. I confirmed that evening that I was pregnant again. As always, Noel was absolutely over the moon. I was also very happy. I had a new outlook on life. It became very important to me that we did everything that we possibly could when we were still able. I refused to take one day for granted. We were lucky because Annie Kate and Aisling were very easy babies, so I was positive that we could more than handle a third.

The morning sickness persisted and looking back, we were comical. The workmen must have thought that we were crazy. Noel and I never mastered the art of curtailing our feelings in public. If we are happy, we are happy and if we are not, then we are simply not. One morning, Noel had a really important meeting to attend at his office. He loaded the children into the car and was all ready to go but I was throwing up in the bathroom. I just couldn't stop throwing up. Noel was getting impatient and yelled from the door for me to hurry up. I went crazy just as the workmen were arriving. I asked them all if they knew of a way to speed up morning sickness. They said nothing. The anger seemed to settle me so we headed to the car. Noel and I were laughing within seconds but it was around that time that he decided to get hand controls for the car and retake his driving test.

During my third pregnancy I remember going for my twenty week scan. The scan revealed two pointers for Downs Syndrome. I panicked a bit because I didn't want the girls to have to deal with anymore. I also debated whether or not to tell Noel because I didn't want to stress him out. Noel however knows me very well and I can never hide anything from him, so I ended up telling him. He told me that if the baby was Downs then it was Downs.

"Downs is not that big a deal," he said.

He truly was not bothered at all. He was obviously still high on life and I decided to join him. I remember feeling at that time that we would have handled a baby with Downs Syndrome just fine.

Mom, Dad, Annie and Neilus arrived early December 2000 to welcome the new baby. Mom and Annie, like all Irish women who visit us, went shopping. They all go crazy shopping, like really crazy, especially since the euro was introduced. Anyway, when I went into labor, Mom and Annie were at the Garden State Plaza Mall. They managed to find a taxi but the driver had very little English and the pair had no idea how to get home. They just knew to make a left at the house with the reindeer. Every second house had reindeer on their front lawn so they spent hours in that taxi. Fortunately, Noel could drive at this point so he drove me to the hospital and decided to attend the birth. This time, Noel really wanted to be there and thank God, the birth was very easy. Sara was born Dec 13th and I felt a huge sense of relief when I first held her. That was a special moment.

When Sara arrived, I was very happy with life. I was delighted to have three healthy babies. They were a joy. Noel used to rush home from work every evening to be with us all. At this stage his MS was visible all the time as he had developed obvious foot drop and everywhere we went it was much easier for him if he was pushing the stroller. Also, his bladder was starting to weaken. His MS was still progressing but we were happy, busy and high on life. If he dipped a lot, he took steroids and every Saturday I gave him the Avonex shot. We were doing all that we could to fight back.

Then two things happened. He got a cane and I got a computer.

Chapter 9

We rang in 2001 with no knowledge that it would prove to be a very difficult year. It is that year that makes me appreciate the good times all the more. In January 2001, Noel bought his first walking cane. Initially it was to help him get to the car in the snow. We bought the cane from Town and Country Pharmacy in Ridgewood. I remember that because of the wonderful service they provided. It was a classy cane. It was black with a silver handle and I was relieved that Noel finally had a cane to help him. I told people that he didn't get it because he had progressed. I insisted that he should have had it years ago just to make life easier. It is clear looking back that he got the cane because he had progressed.

Normally, at that time, when he came home from work in the evenings he would put his cane in the closet. He did not need it around the house initially.

Then in June 2001, my Uncle Neilus was diagnosed with Parkinson's Disease. My family and I were back and forth with e-mail all the time at this point. Neilus had a shake in his right arm for some time, and although everybody hoped and prayed for the best, we were somewhat prepared for bad news. However, the diagnosis was a devastating blow to all of us. It was difficult to believe that Neilus could have Parkinsons, because nobody in our family ever had Parkinsons, and Neilus always epitomized masculine strength, so it just didn't seem right.

Once we confirmed that the diagnosis was correct we had to accept it. I have observed a common thread, not only in my family but also in my dealings with many others. It seems to me that the knee jerk response of people when they hear that a loved one is diagnosed with something like Parkinsons or MS, is to firmly and instantly decide that the loved one has the best possible MS, or the best possible Parkinsons. This is easy to do because there is no map to guide anyone through a linear progression. It was a great relief to me at the time to hear and believe that Neilus had the best possible Parkinsons. As Parkinson's Disease went, Neilus was going to have it very easy. I thought about Neilus all the time that summer and planned a trip home with my girls to be with him.

After my trip home, Mom phoned me to tell me that she found a lump in her breast and her doctor wanted to remove it for a biopsy. She didn't want to mention it when I was home in case it ruined my visit. In September 2001, Mom called me to tell me that she had breast cancer.

She was dreading telling me because I am so far away and we are very close. She and Annie feared that my panic attacks would return. I had learned much about life at this point. Phil's tip to pray served me well. I became Mom's support and told her that we were going to beat it together. Between herself, Annie and I, I assured her that everything would be just fine.

Then, October 2001 came and a very close friend of mine from the Mom's Group at Nativity, told me that she was recently diagnosed with MS. Fortunately for all concerned, it was the best possible MS you could hope for. As MS went, she was going to have it very easy. My friend was thirty at the time. Her two children were very young, and her husband continues to puzzle the rest of us because he tends to her every need. I am certain that his attentive nature has landed many of the other husbands from the group in much trouble over the years.

Growing up, my dad always told me if ever I was down or just plain old angry that I wasn't looking at things right. He used to say that there is good in everything if you look at it right. I now know what he meant. There is much good in everything if you look at it right. I would not wish the good fortune of MS on anyone, but I can clearly see all the good that Noel's MS brought to our family. It has, for example, revealed strengths that he possesses that I may never have noticed otherwise and it has forced us to appreciate every breath. But 2001 tested me, and I really had to squint at times to see any good anywhere in anything.

In the background MS kept creeping up on us. It kept slowly progressing as always.

Our girls were growing up fast. Annie turned three, Aisling turned two and Sara was nearly one. My life was starting to get easy again. They were such fun and great friends and I just loved being with them. They all slept through the night at this stage and I had more mental energy because I too could sleep once again. In November 2001, I started to seriously research MS and Parkinsons on the internet. I really didn't know very much about them at all up to that point so I started reading and reading and reading. It became an obsession. I hated what I read but I couldn't stop.

Initially, the learning curve was very steep because I had to wade through much medical jargon, but I understood it. I was able to piece it all together somehow. The more I read and understood, the easier it was to read and understand more. I firmly concluded that MS really sucks. I didn't share my obsession with Noel. He knew that I was reading about it but he wasn't that interested in it. I concluded that he was smart because why know how awful MS can be when you may luck out and get it easy. The more I read, the more I realized that very few people get MS very easy. It was clear, MS sucks. It was equally clear that Parkinsons sucks and the chances of Neilus having it easy were very slim.

Then came January 2002 and Noel started to slip fast.

Chapter 10

At first I really only noticed his increased dependence on his cane around the house. It was no big deal initially, but I was aware that he was slipping a little. At the time, I was delighted that Mom's breast cancer was the best possible breast cancer there is. She told me that she didn't need a mastectomy, chemotherapy or radiation.

"Mary," she said, "it is only a little nothing."

My bubble didn't last long because I read about breast cancer and called her doctor. I discovered that she had a long road ahead of her but I felt sure that she would get through it.

We spent many hours on the phone back then. When I was growing up, she was always the ultimate optimist grounded in prayer. She is incredibly selfless and always the peacemaker. She was so glad that I didn't flip out. As long as I was okay, she promised that she would be fine. I was more than okay. I guided her through what to expect and all the questions to ask her doctors. I told her how long things should take and how she would feel afterwards. I even told her that she would lose her hair but then told her not to worry about it because it would grow back better.

Mom had the strangest view of her cancer. First, in her mind as always, was the firm belief that God never gives you more than you can handle because God is very good. Second, was sincere gratitude that it was she that had the cancer instead of anybody in her family. She figured that it was much easier to actually deal with it than to watch any of us deal with it. Granted, I would suck at her role, just as I would at Noel's, but still, it made me see why they always got on so well. They share a very similar view of life and faith. In her mind, she was very lucky.

As is tradition in Ireland, her cancer was not discussed much and life went on as normal. I remember phoning home when the family was all gathered shortly before her mastectomy, and nobody seemed to have a care in the world. Mom liked that. Then, when she started her treatment, I heard from friends of mine in nursing that she was the life and soul of the hospital, stunning people with cancer and those working with cancer with her attitude.

After her mastectomy, Mom needed chemotherapy because the cancer had spread to her lymph nodes. She went the whole nine yards. They told her that she would probably feel tired and nauseous after each treatment. She told them her daughter in the States explained it all to her and then she went on to talk nonstop about her three grand daughters. Dad told her that chemotherapy could prove to be a useful diet. She laughed about that. Annie drove five hours to be with her for every treatment and as soon as she was done they would have a three-course meal and hit the shops until they shut. Mom never felt nauseous at all and she didn't lose any weight. She did lose her hair and set a trend with head scarves.

After her chemotherapy, Mom was told that she would have to go to Dublin for radiation therapy. I planned a trip home with my girls to surprise her on completion. As I was planning my trip back to Ireland, Noel was steadily declining in the background. It was spring 2002 and I remember watching him cut the grass. He was no longer able to do it without resting periodically because his legs just kept giving in on him. It was time to confront the fact that Avonex was failing him.

I was not sure at all what to do at this point. Noel realized that he was slipping but as always he was completely fine about it. When I would ask him how he felt, he used to give me the biggest hug and tell me that he was just fine. I pointed out that I noticed that cutting the grass was getting difficult for him and he said that was just the way MS was. He said that he was mentally prepared for the worst and just wanted to enjoy the fact that although he stumbled and had to rest a bit, he was still able to cut the grass. That was a great thing, he claimed. I started to feel very uneasy about my upcoming trip home.

Noel and Mom always had a very special bond. He insisted that I go home for a month to be with her and he promised that he would join us for the last two weeks. I hesitated. I asked him to go and see his neurologist before my flight just to set my mind at ease. He assured me that he was fine but if that was what it took for me to surprise my mom then he would go. Noel went to see his neurologist shortly before my flight home and he was told that he was fine. My mind settled, I figured that I must just have been over reacting seeing as my mind was focused on Mom for so long. I felt so relieved. Thank God everything was okay, I thought.

My three girls and I flew to Dublin late April 2002. The girls are great travelers. I suppose they are just used to it. It is amazing how accommodating people on an airplane are when you have three kids under four. Everybody was more than happy to give us as much room as possible and move to a seat, far, far away. It is better than traveling first class.

My youngest brother Kevin and his wife Lisa, were living in Dublin so we had a royal welcome. Annie was also there to greet us. As always it felt great to be in Ireland. We headed to Kevin and Lisa's house and planned to see Mom in the morning. Word had already slipped out that we had landed and were going to surprise her. I remember thinking that I could just not wait until I would see her in the morning.

As soon as it was morning we went to St. Luke's hospital in Dublin. It was a beautiful morning, really beautiful. It was sunny and warm with a bright, blue sky. I hate hospitals and this one reminded me of an old folks home I worked for in Belfast during my year out from my studies. It had a particular scent that I hated and I just wanted to get Mom out of there.

My children have had a ridiculous fear of elevators for the longest time. I have no idea where they got it from and usually I make them endure the ride, but this was special so we took the stairs. I needed to conserve all of my energy, and climbing a few flights of stairs with three young ones was considered a savings in my book.

I saw Mom. She looked so fresh-faced and she was wearing a head scarf that I had sent her from the states. We were incredibly happy so see each other. She was done! It was over!

Thank God for children. They took our focus and had all sorts of stories for Grandma Maureen. Meanwhile, Granny Annie decided it was time to eat. We all headed for the hospital cafeteria because Mom said that she had many people whom she felt that she had to thank and say goodbye to. I felt so strong every time I looked at her and actually saw her. I prayed that everything would be okay. I wasn't pretending to be strong anymore. I really was strong.

We all started to have fun. The three girls were the life and soul of our fun. From Dublin we headed to Galway and after a stint in Galway with Grandpa Vince we headed to Arranmore. Grandpa Neilus had such a crazy welcome for us all. He had every toy you could imagine for the girls, including a bouncy castle and a swing set. Luckily for me, Annie and Neilus never had a family of their own. I always told them that that was because I needed them more than anyone.

It was immediately obvious to me that Neilus had slipped. His Parkinsons had progressed without question. His shake was now very apparent, but thank God he had the best possible Parkinsons. We all had fun together. It felt so good and we were looking forward to Noel joining us early May.

Noel was finally due to arrive in a couple of days. He called me one night and told me that he was finding it difficult to walk. He assured me that it was no big deal. He explained that his biggest concern was preparing his parents to greet him at the airport in a wheelchair. He figured that he would definitely need a wheelchair on this visit because he was familiar with the distance at the airport. He asked me if I could meet him with his parents to help make light of it all. We were used to wheelchairs from Disney and other parks in the States. I asked him to describe his decline. He told me that he was getting better and starting to feel stronger because his neurologist had given him steroids. He didn't have to say anymore. The fact that he went to his neurologist without me nagging him to death said it all. I told him not to worry about his parents. I assured him that I would organize a fanfare to greet him and with all of the commotion it was possible that his parents would not even notice his wheelchair.

I hung up and could not wait to see him. This time, I even made light of the situation with Mom and Annie. I had toughened up a great deal in the last few years and I was starting to reap the benefits.

Chapter 11

Noel is the only boy of four. He was always the pride and joy of his parents. They never accepted his MS very well by any means. It hit them very hard, especially his mother, Maura. She figured that he had suffered enough in life and for her, his MS was the last straw. She could not stand to think of him slowly deteriorating. She couldn't even pretend that she could. This put a great strain on their relationship because Noel hated to see his mother upset knowing that there was nothing he could do to fix it. Equally, it upset Maura that Noel could not relate to her pain. Noel, I suppose, is a typical man. His way of dealing with something is to provide a solution. His solution for his MS was acceptance and that was not easy for many. When he called his mom to say that he would need a wheelchair at the airport for this visit, I knew that it would deeply upset her. I also knew that no fanfare would hide his wheelchair from her because I understood that she was eagerly waiting to analyze his current condition.

I picked up the phone and called Maura, and as I expected she was very upset. I told her that it wasn't easy but it was important that we all remained calm and strong for Noel. He was genuinely handling the whole thing so well and I really felt that everybody else owed him that. I knew that it wasn't going to be easy on Maura and in many ways it is hardest on her most of all because she is not with him all the time. If you are with somebody with MS constantly, you gradually adjust to their decline. It seems that just being with Noel all the time makes it easier to accept. Distance, however, makes it very difficult and distance also wreaks havoc on an imagination steeped in fear.

Maura and his dad wanted to meet Noel on their own in Dublin with no fanfare. I understood and respected that so we agreed that the girls and I would head to Fahan and meet him at his parent's house after they picked him up. I am very fond of Noel's parents and am grateful that we have a very honest relationship. We always feel comfortable speaking our mind.

As soon as I saw Noel, it was instantly clear that he had slipped. He was now completely dependent on his cane and the distance that he could walk had greatly diminished. Also, his bladder was very weak. But Noel was high on life. He was so happy to see the girls and me, and he had many stories about traveling with a disability.

Noel's pet hate in life is people's lack of consideration for others. Couple that with a disdain for incompetence and add a dash of impatience to understand why it was funny to hear how he had to wait on the plane for so long after everybody else disembarked because somebody forgot to get him a wheelchair. Noel learns fast. As soon as we got back to the States he bought his own chair. He decided that he never wanted to wait for a wheelchair ever again.

We had a lot of fun in Fahan. We knew that it was difficult for his parents but I think that everybody made the best of the situation. After Fahan, we traveled to Galway, and before we knew it we were all back in New Jersey.

Soon it was June 2002, and Noel continued to decline. He could no longer cut the front lawn at all and to do the back he needed to rest four or five times. It was very difficult to watch him but the way he handled it was literally beyond belief. He never ever complained. He was always so happy and fun to be with. I kept my vow to be strong for him but I confess that I found it difficult at times.

As soon as he would leave for work in the morning I used to gather the children and pray. It really did keep me sane. The only time I felt truly at peace was when I prayed. The children loved it. I suppose that children sense everything, especially ill-hidden tension. They liked it when I was calm. That is what prayer did for me, it always calmed me. Obviously, I couldn't pray all day as I had much to tend to. The children had classes and I needed Wednesday mornings at Nativity.

Many from the Mom's Group were deeply concerned for me at this point, but I was strong. I had a coping mechanism in place. Also,

I had hope. I was starting to read about people with MS on the internet who had taken their health into their own hands. They described how they felt the medical community and MS societies had failed them. Some were on bee stings, others were on a particular diet and others were using histamine. There seemed to be a whole array of options to explore.

It was very clear to me at this point that the Avonex was not working for Noel. I read everything about Avonex and even Biogen advised people to come off it if they started to progress rapidly. I told Noel what I thought, but Noel told me that he had a problem believing me because I was not a neurologist. True, he had a very valid point. Noel really liked his neurologist at this stage and felt that he was getting the best possible treatment. He explained that he had a neurologist so that the neurologist could tell him what drugs to take and when to come off them. That was his neurologist's job, he insisted.

Noel honestly felt that it was futile to waste valuable time chasing a pipe dream. He told me that people must go crazy trying to fight MS. He explained to me that it made much more sense to him to maximize every second he had with his family. He vowed that he would never make MS his life or undertake a quest to find a cure or indulge in any form of quackery. He insisted that he would let his neurologist decide what was best for him on every turn and he told me quite firmly to just leave it at that. He really wanted to keep going at full speed for as long as possible. He asked me to accept his condition and to just make the most of whatever we had.

I love his strength and acceptance. He holds an unnerving conviction that he will pass the test regardless of circumstance and it is admirable. But, I could not let it be. I told him that if I had MS, I would wear a histamine patch, eat everything raw and despite a ridiculous bee phobia, I would sting myself daily. I told him that I would fight with everything I had. I told him that I really wished that it were me that had MS instead of him because I would fight hard and beat it.

It is silly what people wish for. I mean, if I was granted a wish at that point in time it would have been for me to have MS instead of Noel. How crazy a wish is that? I really wish that nobody in the world had MS at all, ever. Really, how could my mother ever have been grateful that she had cancer instead of anyone else? It just doesn't make any sense to me. I would be grateful if nobody in the world had cancer, ever. That would be good. But, if I had MS I repeated, at least I would fight and I would really fight.

Noel laughed and told me that was why he was so glad that I didn't have MS. It was better for us that it was him who had to deal with it instead of me in his mind. He told me that if I had MS I would turn it into an unhealthy obsession.

"Let's just enjoy every second of every day we have together," he used to say.

I was never quite sure if his coping mechanism for dealing with MS was a form of denial or a genuine gift of grace. As more time passes I am pretty convinced that it is the gift of grace.

Every morning Noel would go to work and I would pray with the children to calm myself and in my spare time I used to read about MS on the internet. I could not let it be. I just had to fight, so I read and I read and I read. It was apparent that along with sucking, MS is incredibly elusive. It is true that what works for one person may not work for somebody else. For me to confront Noel again I needed better than that. I needed something that was working across the board. I suppose I needed a miracle.

I kept telling the Mom's Group that there had to be somebody somewhere who knew how to treat MS effectively. I remember they used to nod sympathetically at me. I am sure that they thought that I was losing my mind but I knew that I wasn't. I was just searching. Then one morning I found what I was looking for.

I often look back on that morning in early August 2002. I was very tired and I had shut myself off from the Mom's Group to make time for my search. I started to skip our Wednesday morning sessions. Many from the group phoned me daily even when I didn't return calls. They just persisted and often called round to surprise me. They were always more than welcome, I was just preoccupied at the time because there was so much to read.

One particular morning Noel went to work and I prayed. His balance was absolutely dreadful. He could hardly get off the couch without three or four heaves and when he finally managed it, he often fell over. I had plans to buy him a walker for the house and I was seriously considering moving our bedroom downstairs because it was a nightmare to watch him climb the stairs at night. Things really were very grim. However, as always, Noel's spirits were great and he was quite prepared for a permanent wheelchair.

"A wheelchair is no big deal," he said.

I laugh about this now because it is a little bit funny. It used to take me so long to calm myself before leaving the house for various children classes that I often misplaced things, especially my keys. I used to lose my keys three to four times a day. Like many in Ireland, I was trained at a young age to pray to St. Anthony if ever I lost anything because he is the saint in charge of lost and found. Amazingly, it often worked for me. Overtired and leaving the house with the three children I used to automatically ask St. Anthony to help me find my keys and I would find them. This particular morning on finding my keys I laughed and said to the children that it would be great if St. Anthony would invest his time more wisely and find what I really needed. I really needed to find the right treatment for Noel because I was more than convinced that the Avonex was completely failing him, even harming him. So, I asked St. Anthony to find me the right treatment for Noel.

Now, here is a choice moment—if by any possible chance I had St. Anthony's ear, talk about wasting my moment. It is again like the wasted wish, wishing that I had MS instead of Noel. I mean honestly, if I thought that the guy was listening at all I would have asked him to find me a cure to put an end to all of the craziness. I don't know if St. Anthony ever heard me but I like to imagine that he did. It would be a great story if he really did. I have since asked him to find a cure and although he hasn't found one yet, I will keep asking.

I do know for certain that I was thinking of buying a walker for Noel at the time and I was trying to remember for days where I bought his cane because I liked the service they provided. I had basically given up on remembering and had intended to shop elsewhere that afternoon. It was that day on logging out of the internet that I noticed a pop up window with the address and phone number of Town and Country Pharmacy in Ridgewood. That was the name and number I was trying to remember and find for days because that was where we bought his cane. I dialed the number immediately to inquire about various walking aids for Noel and the owner John, answered the phone.

I remembered that when we bought Noel's cane that they were very helpful in Town and Country. I remembered feeling that they just seemed to go that extra mile for people. It is not nice to have to buy a cane but they made it seem okay. I recognized John's voice when he answered the phone. I just said that my husband had MS and John interrupted me. I wanted to thank him for the wonderful service he provides and ask him about walkers and all different types of walking aides. I knew that he would be able to tell me a great deal about them and I also knew that if he didn't stock exactly what I needed that he would know a man who did. Anyway, I never had any of that conversation with him. The first thing that he asked me on hearing that my husband had MS was whether or not my husband was taking LDN. I said no and I asked him what LDN was.

He told me about a customer and friend of his who had a website at http://www.goodshape.net/. Mr. Goodshape was married to Polly, he continued and he told me that Polly had very severe MS. Her MS was progressing rapidly he said, but by all accounts it seemed to have completely stopped since she started taking LDN two years previously. John told me that he compounded the LDN for Polly and although he confessed that he didn't know a great deal about the drug, he did know that it was a safe bet because it had no known side effects. He said that he thought LDN may be worth a shot. He told me that Mr. Goodshape had a lot more information on his website.

John also explained to me that Noel might have difficulty getting a prescription for the drug because it was not listed for use with MS. He said that some people who could not persuade their neurologists, asked their Primary Care Physicians to prescribe the drug for them off label because it was already FDA approved at a much higher dose for heroin addicts. Before I hung up, John finished by telling me that if I needed any help in convincing Noel's neurologist to prescribe LDN, that he was more than willing to help me in any way possible. I deeply appreciated his concern and willingness to help. Once again he went the extra mile. I decided to investigate and I could not believe what I read.

Even for an optimist, it sounded too good to be true.

Chapter 12

I logged onto the internet and went to Goodshape's site. There was much information on the benefits of histamine but I had already presented histamine as an option to Noel and I knew that he wasn't interested. I was specifically looking for information on LDN and then I found it. Goodshape had a link to the LDN MS page. This is the first thing I read and I could not take it in initially.

"Clinically the results are strongly suggestive of efficacy. 98 to 99% of people treated with LDN experience no more disease progression, whether the disease category is relapsing-remitting or chronic progressive. Dr. Bihari has more than seventy people with MS in his practice and all are stable over an average of three years. The original patient on LDN for MS, now on it for seventeen years, has not had an attack or disease progression for twelve years since the one missed month that led to an attack.

In addition, 2,000 or more people with MS have been prescribed LDN by their family MDs or their neurologists based on what they have read on the LDN website or heard about in internet chat rooms focused on MS. Many such patients with MS, not under Dr. Bihari's care, use the e-mail link on the LDN website to ask questions. Many prescribing physicians do not generally know about LDN.

Only once has a patient reported disease progression while on LDN. In this case, it showed itself five days after he had started the drug. The onset of the episode had apparently preceded the start of LDN.

In addition to the apparent ability of LDN to stop disease progression, approximately two-thirds of MS patients starting LDN have some symptomatic improvement generally apparent within the first few days. There are two types of such improvement.

One is reduction in spasticity when this is present, sometimes allowing easier ambulation when spasticity in the legs has been a prominent element of a patient's difficulty in walking or standing. This is unlikely to represent a direct effect of LDN on the disease process, but rather reduction in the irritability in nervous tissue surrounding plaques. Endorphins have been shown to reduce irritability of nervous tissue, e.g., by reducing seizures in patients with epilepsy.

The other area of symptomatic improvement in some patients is a reduction in MS-related fatigue. This is, also, not likely due to a direct effect on the MS disease process, but rather an indirect one caused by restoration of normal endorphin levels improving energy.

Patients who are in the midst of an acute exacerbation when they start LDN have generally shown rapid resolution of the attack. In two patients, chronic visual impairment due to old episodes of optic neuritis has shown fluctuating improvement.

It should be emphasized that in spite of the plentitude of clinical experience described above, in the absence of a formal clinical trial of LDN in MS, these results cannot be considered scientific, but rather anecdotal. A clinical trial, preferably by a pharmaceutical company with some experience with MS, is clearly needed to determine whether these results can be replicated. If they can be, they are likely to lead to widespread use of this extremely non-toxic drug in the treatment of MS."

That was my starting point. At this point I was well aware of the chances of standard MS drugs slowing the progression of relapsing remitting MS only, and none of them came remotely close to this. I mean, this was saying that LDN does not slow the progression, it actually stops MS from progressing 98-99% of the time regardless of the type of MS. It was unbelievable. I instantly decided that I didn't want to know anything more about LDN until I thoroughly investigated the doctor making these claims, Dr. Bernard Bihari. I also wanted to quickly figure out who was profiting from the website advertising these bold claims.

I performed an internet wide search on Dr. Bernard Bihari that led me to the home page of the LDN webpage. I laughed because it took me a while to travel that circle. I noticed that Dr. Bihari's Cirriculum Vitae (CV) was part of the site so I looked and I thought that it read very well. It said that he achieved his MD from Harvard and it stated his New York State Medical License Number 088158. I used that number to verify part of his CV with the New York State Education Department. I found his record and it read

Name : BIHARI BERNARD
Address : NEW YORK, NY
Profession : MEDICINE
License No: 088158
Date of Licensure : 09/07/62
Additional Qualification : A - Certified to practice acupuncture
Status : REGISTERED Registered through last day of : 10/05
Medical School: HARVARD UNIVERSITY
Degree Date : 06/13/1957

I continued to investigate and read on his CV that he was board certified since 1970. I confirmed that information with the American Board of Psychiatry and Neurology. His CV also stated that he was an attending physician at Beth Israel Medical Center in New York so I phoned Beth Medical and confirmed that information. I concluded that it was difficult to believe that Dr. Bihari was a quack because his credentials were solid.

Then I checked out the website itself to see who was sponsoring it. I was again impressed that it was a non-profit website . I read the following

"This website is sponsored by Advocates For Therapeutic Immunology. The purpose of this website is to provide information to patients and physicians about important therapeutic breakthroughs in advanced medical immunology. The authors of this site do not profit from the sale of LDN or from website traffic, and are in no way associated with any pharmaceutical manufacturer or pharmacy."

I became convinced that Dr. Bihari was not a quack nor was he out to make a fast dollar. I was intrigued to say the least so I decided to find out what LDN actually was.

I learned that LDN stood for Low Dose Naltrexone. Naltrexone hydrochloride is a white powder chemical compound. It is a drug that is listed in the Physician's Desk Reference (PDR) and is an approved treatment for substance use disorders such as heroin addiction. Since it is listed in the PDR, doctors may use their own judgment in deciding whether to prescribe naltrexone to other individuals, such as those with Multiple Sclerosis. Naltrexone is marketed as Revia, and although it is primarily a narcotic antagonist, it has also been shown to reduce craving and consumption for some patients who are alcohol dependent. The FDA approved standard dose given to patients with a substance abuse problem is 50mg naltrexone.

At first I didn't understand what the connection could possibly be between a drug used for substance abuse and MS. Then it became clear. There really isn't one. Low Dose Naltrexone is not supposed to serve the same purpose as naltrexone. At a low dose, 4.5mg, Dr. Bihari was using LDN to boost the immune systems of his patients. Now that flies in the face of conventional MS thinking because the standard MS medications work on suppressing the immune system based on the theory that people with MS have an overactive immune system. Dr. Bihari was challenging all conventional views of MS by trying to boost the immune system as opposed to suppressing it. I was very curious what prompted his thinking so I read more and I dug deeper. I think that my findings make an interesting story.

Dr. Bihari's early work consisted of helping those afflicted with drug and alcohol abuse in New York City. From there, in the 1980s, his work extended to the HIV and AIDS community. It is during this time that he discovered the therapeutic uses of LDN for HIV and AIDS. From what I know of the man, I believe that his heart lies in helping the AIDS epidemic and that he stumbled into helping the MS community serendipitously.

In 1988, his daughter's best friend was diagnosed with MS and because Dr. Bihari had seen the capability of LDN to boost the immune system in his HIV and AIDS patients he prescribed 3mg LDN for his daughter's friend. He believed HIV, AIDS and MS had one thing in common, and that was that they were diseases based on disturbed immune systems. It was more than plausible in Dr. Bihari's mind that LDN would work for MS seeing as it was showing great promise in HIV and AIDS patients in his practice.

His daughter's friend was twenty-two years old in 1988 and there was absolutely no treatment whatsoever for MS. Dr. Bihari prescribed 3mg LDN for her and she took it for five years with no progression. Then, she went out of state and her LDN supply ran out. She felt so good, she figured that she didn't need it anymore, so she stopped taking it. Within a month or so her MS started to flare up again so she immediately resumed LDN treatment. To this day she takes LDN and she has not progressed. She is the first MS patient on this treatment and a remarkable testimony to its benefits.

For many years since 1988, Dr. Bihari dedicated himself to the AIDS crisis, but through word of mouth the potential that LDN had for MS spread, and he was contacted by more and more people suffering with MS. At first the word spread very slowly. By the time I actually followed his story through, and picked up the phone to speak with him, he had less than eighty patients with MS, but they were all stable regardless of the type of MS they were diagnosed with.

I remember working up the nerve to call Dr. Bihari. His address and phone number were part of his CV that was posted on the LDN site. Noel was at work and my three girls were napping. I had no idea what to expect but I was more than pleasantly surprised.

Chapter 13

My first surprise was that Dr. Bihari actually answered the phone himself. I introduced myself and explained that I had been reading about his work on the internet and that I just wanted to talk to him about it before presenting it all to Noel. Dr. Bihari was very friendly. I was honest with him and I told him that it read far too good to be true. I explained that I didn't want to play on Noel's emotions and that I had to be very certain of my information before I even thought about raising Noel's hopes. Dr. Bihari completely understood and proceeded to assure me that all I read was true. He started at the very beginning and explained everything to me in terms that I could understand. His manner was laid back and very relaxed. He was very easy to talk with and listen to and I felt his compassion. He told me about his work in the AIDS and HIV community but I wasn't interested in any of that at the time. I just wanted to know about LDN and MS.

Dr. Bihari told me that he believed that everybody with an autoimmune disorder has low levels of endorphins. Before he explained what endorphins were he told me what exactly an autoimmune disease is. He said that the word "auto" is the Greek word for self. The immune system is a complicated network that normally works to defend the body and eliminate infections, but if a person has an autoimmune disease, the immune system mistakenly attacks itself, targeting the cells, tissues and organs of a person's own body. There are many different autoimmune diseases, and they can each affect the body in different ways. For example, the autoimmune reaction is directed against the brain and spinal cord in Multiple Sclerosis, and the gut in Crohn's disease.

I had read on the internet that there are many theories as to what MS actually is and it is even debated as to whether or not it is autoimmune. Also, the definitions and naming of various types and stages of MS is highly debated. Everything about MS is debated. It is incredibly elusive. That is what makes it even more frustrating, but Dr. Bihari firmly believes that MS is an autoimmune disease. He believes that is why LDN stops it in its tracks.

Dr. Bihari continued and explained to me that just as the sex hormone testosterone controls sexual function, so too do endorphins control and regulate the immune system. Dr. Bihari said that endorphins are produced nightly between the hours of 9:00 p.m. and 2:00 a.m. and that 4.5mg LDN, if taken between these hours, triples endorphin production bringing the levels up to normal. He claimed that if endorphin production is regulated, they would be able to control and regulate the immune system. Hence, the immune system would no longer be able to attack itself. He told me that was why none of his MS patients progressed. It was that simple.

"It is not a cure for MS," he insisted. He stated that LDN would only remove the last three months worth of damage if Noel was lucky, but it seemed to be universal in stopping disease progression.

That was a great deal of information for me to take in at the time and in my mind it still sounded too good to be true. I proceeded to tell Dr. Bihari about my Uncle Neilus and his Parkinsons. To my amazement, Dr. Bihari told me that although Parkinsons was medically documented with unknown etiology, he believed that Parkinsons was also an autoimmune disease. He told me that because of his success with HIV, AIDS and MS, he started branching out in to a whole spectrum of what he considered to be autoimmune diseases. He explained that he was very thankful for the internet because it made it possible for him to reach so many more people than ever before. He was excited and he told me that he had three Parkinsons patients on LDN for over a year and that although it was too early for him to say for sure that it worked, he assured me that it looked very promising. If nothing else, he insisted LDN was worth a try for Parkinsons based on the fact that there are no side effects and it is a very inexpensive therapy.

Our conversation continued to naturally flow. It was a very long phone call. I think that I spoke with Dr. Bihari for over forty-five minutes in total. I asked him about breast cancer and I explained to him that my Mom had a recent mastectomy and had just finished her chemotherapy and radiation therapy. Again he was most eager to share. He told me that he and his wife were actually taking LDN themselves for about ten years to prevent cancer as it was very prevalent in both of their families. He told me that he had twenty women with breast cancer on LDN for five years and that all were still in remission. He said that typically half of them would have had a reoccurrence by now without LDN. It really was difficult to believe what I was hearing but I knew by talking with him that he really believed it and it seemed that he had great reason to do so.

I thanked him at the end of our call and asked him if I should pay him. He refused payment. He said that he was delighted that I had found the website on LDN and that he was positive that LDN would greatly help my family. He explained that any doctor could prescribe LDN for his or her patients and he told me that he was delighted to share his information with me and he wished me well. He just asked that should my family decide to take LDN, that I would make sure that it was compounded as described on the LDN website. He assured me that it was an easy thing to do and that any compounding pharmacy could do it if instructed properly but it was important that it was compounded correctly for it to work.

I hung up and I sat quiet for a bit. I decided not to say anything to anyone just yet because I needed it to sink in. I needed to read more.

I believed Dr. Bihari at this point but I wanted to hear what others were saying. I was well aware of my ability to be overly optimistic and I wanted to keep myself in check. I had to be really sure of everything before speaking with Noel, Neilus and Mom.

I called my brother Phil that evening. He was an established doctor at this stage so I asked him if LDN could possibly do Noel any harm. To my amazement Phil was most interested in my findings. Phil specializes in NaProTECHNOLOGY, a new reproductive and gynecologic science which has been developed at the Pope Paul VI Institute for the Study of Human Reproduction. The Institute has created a standardized modification of the Billings Ovulation Method and called it the Creighton Model FertilityCare System. Anyway, Phil told me that they use LDN at much higher doses to boost fertility for some couples. He believes that LDN somehow boosts fertility by boosting endorphins, and he assured me that at 4.5mg it would do no harm to Noel. Phil told me that LDN for MS was completely in line with the first guiding principle of medicine according to Hippocrates, "Primum non nocere" or "First do no harm."

Phil completely reassured me that I was on the right track so I continued to investigate. The only internet message board that discussed LDN at the time was Goodshape's, so I decided to thoroughly investigate his site.

Chapter 14

A message board is a meeting place on the internet where people with a common interest can share their views and experience. To be honest, at the time, I thought that such boards were only for people who couldn't relate in the real world. I thought that internet "chat rooms" were only for people who needed to hide behind a computer screen. But I was intrigued by the Goodshape site because John, the pharmacist from Town and Country in Ridgewood knew him. I lurked for a bit and just read what people had to say. I had friends whom I could talk to if I needed to, but the internet provided something different. It provided an instant community of people in a similar position to mine, all fighting the same enemy.

When I first started posting on Goodshape's site I did feel like "Mary no friends" because it was clear that my friends and family could not understand the issues that these people behind the screen could. I actually started to enjoy conversing with Goodshape and members of his site. I looked forward to getting home in the evenings to hear what was new or who had responded to my latest query. It was addictive. I heard many stories about LDN. They were all positive and I admired Goodshape for hosting the group. I even related to his circumstance as he too was fighting for his spouse whom he loved more than anything in the whole world. Polly had been on LDN for two years at this time and she had not progressed despite her chronic diagnosis.

Goodshape wrote that he was also taking LDN as a cancer preventative and many people from the board shared heart wrenching stories that could only have been true.

Things were really happening on the Goodshape board. People with MS had hope and they inspired me so I told them my story. I told them that I was happily married to a headstrong man who had a solid conviction that he would carry his cross his way, with pride, and whose latest at the time was to explain to me that the best anyone in life can hope for is the ability to play out their hand with dignity. I shared with them that I had three children under four and that I was convinced of the merits of LDN but knew that I would have a difficult job convincing Noel to even think about it. I asked for help and I was inundated with positive support and creative ideas. I could not believe the accuracy with which these strangers understood my predicament and I was astounded at their eagerness to help a complete stranger. I have to say I was very moved.

They forewarned me of potential nightmare dealings with neurologists and doctors but assured me that the fight was worth it in the end. LDN is the best possible treatment for MS was always the bottom line and they insisted that I never gave up.

I dug some more because I could not help but think that if LDN was so great, then why on earth was it such a secret. I questioned why Noel's neurologist didn't know about this? After all, he attended most of the MS meetings in New York along with the best MS experts in the world. It seemed logical to assume that if there was anything in LDN then he would know about it. But I deduced that if Noel's neurologist did know about LDN, Noel would have been on it, so I figured that Noel's neurologist was not aware of LDN or if he was aware of it, then it was obvious that he was not convinced of its merits. I also questioned why in the world nothing was published about this. I still question that but I don't understand the mechanics of publishing in the medical world. I can only assume that it is not very easy for a cheap drug with no side effects and outrageous promise to get published. It was evident that I had more loose ends to tie up before sharing with family and friends because I knew that I had to be prepared to answer the obvious questions.

I posted my concerns on Goodshape's site and the plot started to thicken and my blood started to boil. Initially, I refused to believe that the world was so corrupt. I refused to believe what I read and part of me still does. A big part of me still cannot buy into this theory that is now believed by many to be true.

It was strongly suggested that the reason LDN had not hit the masses was because the drug companies dishing out the expensive drugs to MS patients stood to lose far too much money. It was spelled out to me that they make a nice profit tending to MS victims and that they were acting on their interests behind the scenes. It was strongly implied that the MS drug companies were actively preventing LDN from hitting the masses. Granted MS therapies are expensive and hence lucrative. Avonex is about $1100 a month compared to $35 maximum a month for LDN, but I still didn't buy into this theory because I felt that it was based on paranoia. Maybe at first I did because I wanted somebody to blame, but as soon as I thought about it in depth I rejected it.

I immediately understood why Dr. Bihari had problems getting the drug into a scientific trial in the US. It made business sense to me. LDN is a cheap drug, it is already FDA approved at ten times the dose, so it holds no monetary incentive for any pharmaceutical or U.S. Government body to run with it. Actually, the U.S. Government would save millions in the long run if even one tenth of what Dr. Bihari claims to be true was in fact true, because more people would be able to work and hence require less from the state. Corporate America however has a short term view of profit and works against the potential of a cheap drug despite the hope it holds for its citizens. That is a sad and tragic reality. But, were the big bad profit crazy drug companies actually actively stopping LDN getting out there? I didn't and I still don't believe that.

The problem I have with that theory is that the LDN community then and although bigger now, is still far too small. It is not big or scary enough yet to make any drug company take it seriously.

As far as I could see, in 2002, there were a handful of LDN advocates who saw LDN work. MS however is very elusive, so the same amount of people could just as easily have been saying that the best way to stop MS progress is to pat your head and rub your tummy three times daily. The enigmatic world of MS provides a fertile breeding ground for quackery.

With regard to reaching the masses with LDN though, I firmly believe that there is no bad guy actively trying to prevent it from happening. I can see how the good guys, such as the MS societies, whose duty it is to help people with MS could be perceived as the bad guys simply because they openly want nothing to do with LDN. However, I believe that the problem with getting anybody to seriously investigate the potential of LDN, particularly in the U.S. comes down to two major things. It lacks financial incentive and equally it lacks credibility. It is too simple a theory, too ridiculous to believe. I mean, even to me, an optimist by nature, with my back against the wall, it was unbelievable.

Today the whole problem with LDN outside of the U.S. in my mind is actually credibility more than anything else.

When I look at the situation in Ireland, I see that the Government pays for all of the expensive MS medications for each person who decides to take them. In Ireland, 6,000 people have MS and about 2,000 of them use a standard MS therapy. Anybody can do the math, 1,200 Euro a month per person versus 30 Euro a month. Of course the Irish Government would prefer to pay for the LDN monthly and have less people dependent on them. They have been presented with a proposal to do a trial on LDN for MS and stand to save millions yearly. The only reason they did not set up a trial on receipt of the proposal has to be credibility (although a skeptic would question whether or not the Government is in bed with the pharmaceutical companies).

An LDN trial requires a leap of faith because the governments don't want to risk funding an actual trial despite the potential it holds for future savings, not to mention future lives.

Anyway, to get back to August 2002, I had reached a point where I felt that I had thoroughly investigated LDN and I decided that it was time to present the information to Noel.

Chapter 15

I think that the best definition of love that I ever heard came from Chris Rock, an American comedian. He said that unless you have thought about murder then you have never been in love.

In August 2002, it is safe to say that Noel and I fell deeply in love. ADP was still reeling from the effects of the terrorist attack on the Twin Towers on September 11th 2001. Every month there were more and more cutbacks so Noel's job was not secure and the prospect of us having to move back to Ireland became very real. Neither of us wanted to move because New Jersey had become our home. We loved all that it had to offer, especially for our children. We just love the way of life and the positive openness of the people. Also, we have a wonderful network of friends with whom we have a lot of fun.

In the midst of all the work stress, the onslaught of Noel's MS continued. It was relentless. Also, the steroids started to lose their magic. Noel developed a level of immunity to steroids. Since then, I have learned that this is quite common.

I remember one evening Noel commented that his worst symptom without a doubt was his weak bladder. His balance was dreadful and I remember I could hear his left leg drag on the carpet when he walked around the house with his cane. He also fell quite a bit and he had great difficulty getting up again. When he slept, his legs twitched every couple of minutes and I remember too, that he used to exercise his hands more. It was apparent that his hands were starting to be affected ever so slightly.

But, as the month passed things became even worse than that. MS stole our ability to be intimate. That put a great strain on our relationship because there are times when we rely on intimacy to communicate. There are no words for some situations. Overall, things were very tense.

One day late August, Noel came home from work. He grabbed a beer and as always he spent the first half an hour rolling around the floor playing with the children. I told him that we needed to talk.

I think that everyone hates hearing those words, especially after a hostile day at work, so Noel ignored me. So, I just started to talk. I told him all about LDN as he wrestled with the children. He said nothing, so I told him it all again. He still said nothing and once again I repeated my thoughts. He finally looked at me and asked me where I found all of my information. He was visibly annoyed at my persistence. I told him about all of my virtual friends in cyberspace and as I had expected he thought that I had lost my mind. I then told him about Dr. Bihari and the phone call I had with him. Noel said that if there was any truth in what I was saying then his neurologist would know about it. I explained that it was quite possible that his neurologist may not have heard about it. I told him that LDN was relatively new for MS and not clinically proven but it was cheap with no side effects, so in my book we had nothing to lose by trying it.

In Noel's mind he had everything to lose he said because it would just be the start of a million different goose chases I would send him on in search of a non-existent cure. He figured it best to nip all of the nonsense in the bud and just enjoy whatever time he had doing whatever he could do. He told me that he understood that it was difficult for me but that I really had to accept his MS and face the fact that things were only going to get a whole lot worse. I was livid and he became livid. I really wanted to kill him and that was mutual. Without question, Chris Rock would have considered us very much in love.

I explained to Noel that just as he wanted me to accept his decline with grace, I wanted him to fight back with everything he had. We were head to head and neither of us was willing to give in. It was too important from both perspectives to budge on this one. It was a very tough situation.

During this time a very good friend of mine from the Mom's Group, Rachel, was preparing to move to Ohio. Her husband was having difficulty finding work in New Jersey and he wanted to move back to his roots. Rachel didn't want to move and she was very stressed out at the time. Actually, it is amazing the effect that September 11th had on many of the Mom's Group and their families. As a group we became tighter than ever.

I remember I called over to Tia the morning after I told Noel about LDN, and Rachel was there. I think most of the Mom's Group turn to Tia in a crisis. She is very warm and non-judgmental. That makes her an easy person to confide in. The three of us are very close so I told them both the whole story. They knew something was up with me for a while but I will never forget their faces. They really didn't know what to make of the LDN story. I will always love them because they went with me blindly. Even though they probably thought that I had lost my mind, they just took my children and told me to go and do whatever I had to do. They told me to follow through with my instincts and not to worry about the children. I left my little ones with them and I went home and logged on to the internet to e-mail a letter to Noel.

I told him that I loved him. I explained that I was worn out and could not stand fighting with him any longer. It was exhausting. I told him that the decision to try LDN had to be his decision because he was the one with MS. I pointed out that I didn't want to stress him out any more. I wrote that if he didn't want to take LDN, then he didn't have to. I told him that I was done arguing and I asked him what he wanted for dinner.

That is something that MS taught me. It is now very important to me not to waste time fighting or arguing. I used to be able to hold a grudge for a good week or so but now I can hardly last a day. We always make a point to end our day on a good note. As I said earlier, I would not wish MS on anyone, but it has given us a rare appreciation of every breath and taught us how to really enjoy the moment, and that is quite a nice way to live. Anyway, Noel replied instantly and said that he wanted shepherd's pie for dinner and added that he had an appointment with his neurologist the following week. He told me that he wanted to try one more blast of steroids. He said that I could accompany him if I so wished and that I could ask his neurologist what he thought about LDN. Noel explained that if his neurologist gave it the go ahead then he would try it.

So, I had a window and I was back in the game. All I had to do was convince Noel's neurologist of the merits of LDN.

I was excited and I called Tia and Rachel. Being familiar with Noel, they really thought that my excitement was premature but kept encouraging me to continue. I spent days preparing for that appointment with Noel's neurologist. I called John from Town and Country Pharmacy to ask for his help. John assured me that he would send Noel's neurologist everything he had on LDN and he did. By the time the appointment came I was more than ready. I will never forget that consultation with Noel's neurologist in September 2002.

I dropped my children off with Tia and Rachel at Tia's house and I met Noel in the waiting room of the neurologist's office. I had a folder under my arm filled with papers that made Noel glare at me on arrival and question what on earth I was planning to do. I told him I was certain that his neurologist would prove difficult so I had to take a couple of printouts in case I forgot to say something. This made Noel very angry. He told me outright not to embarrass him by harassing his neurologist. I laughed nervously and assured him that I would be on my best behavior. Noel eyeballed me and told me that it was not a game. I assured him that a game was the last thing I would compare our situation to. Just then, Noel was called in and I followed. We both sat in the neurologist's office.

As always, the appointment started with the neurological exam. I am sure that this exam reveals something, but Noel literally staggered into the office with his cane, which he didn't have on his previous visit. From my perspective, not knowing anything about how these exams work, it seemed to me that because Noel could still stretch out his arms and touch his nose it was deduced that there had been no change in him. Obviously the tests are more thorough than I give them credit for, but I couldn't believe that it was decided that he had not progressed.

I was starting to twitch myself at this point but I said nothing. The neurologist asked Noel what the problem was and Noel replied that he was feeling a bit weaker than usual and felt that he may need another blast of steroids. The neurologist proceeded to write the standard prescription and Noel started to get ready to leave. Then I asked politely if I could say something.

They both looked at each other and then they looked at me. I was tired, desperate, obsessed and even out of order, because the neurologist did everything by the book and to step outside of that book leaves the guy open to all sorts of liability claims.

However, I said that I was delighted that Noel could still touch his nose but pointed out that I was concerned because he could no longer cut the front grass, climb the stairs or get off the couch without falling over. I said that I was also concerned that he was taking a medication for relapsing remitting MS when it was clear that he had progressive MS and I stated very clearly that Avonex was drastically failing him.

The neurologist asked me to describe Noel's decline. I gave a blow by blow account of his rapidly decreasing level of functionality. The neurologist genuinely appreciated the insight, and then suggested that perhaps Noel should come off the Avonex and start a daily injection of Copaxone instead. Noel was not a bit pleased. He glared at me and a white rim started to form around his tightly clenched mouth. I continued.

I told the neurologist that Copaxone was also only for relapsing remitting MS. I then showed him a number of printouts from the drug companies all stating that their medications were all only for relapsing remitting MS. I even highlighted the printed probability of them working on that type of MS and the lists of side effects they presented. I looked the neurologist in the eye and asked him if he honestly thought any of them worth our while considering our circumstance. I said that our situation was desperate and that I wanted him to prescribe LDN for Noel. Then I asked him if he had read the literature forwarded by John from Town and Country Pharmacy.

The neurologist sat down and asked me to take a seat. He told me that I was obviously under a great deal of stress and that there were professional people who could help me work through my grief. Noel could not hold back any longer and apologized to his neurologist on my behalf. Noel looked at me and told me that I really needed to speak to someone and work out my issues. I looked at them both calmly and agreed that it was quite possible that I did in fact need counseling. Without a doubt that was possible. I mean, once again, Noel's neurologist was simply going by the book, but I refused to accept that. I told them that I would look into therapy if it meant that they would just listen to me. I thanked them calmly for their concern and proceeded.

When I finished the LDN theory, the neurologist raised his eyebrows at me and reminded me of all the MS meetings he attended. He told me that LDN had not gone through any scientific trial and if there was anything at all worth knowing about LDN, then he would know about it. I then asked him outright if it could possibly do Noel any harm. He shrugged and said that he couldn't see what possible harm it could cause. I told him that we at least agreed on something and I asked him to work with me. I asked him, seeing as we both agreed that it could do no harm, would he prescribe it. Noel was fit to kill me at this point. The neurologist thought about it for a brief moment and then he wrote a script for 3mg LDN. He also wrote a script for Copaxone, and finished the one he started for steroids. I have learned since then that it is common practice for neurologists to put their chronic MS patients on MS medicines that have only been tested on relapsing remitting MS. This is done because many neurologists feel that it is the best interest of the patient. I should also point out that many people with primary progressive MS are very grateful for that.

Noel and I left the office in complete silence and we drove home separately. I thought that the meeting went as well as could have been expected. We had the script so Noel could start LDN if he so wished.

I got home and Noel was irate. He was so annoyed that I would try to tell his neurologist how to treat him. I knew that it was time to be quiet. He was very, very angry with me. For the rest of the day it was all picture and no sound in the Bradley house.

Chapter 16

I remember the date of that appointment with Noel's neurologist because it was September 11th 2002. A good friend of ours lost her husband in the World Trade Center the year before and a gang of us from the Mom's Group had planned to meet at the Nativity Church for the memorial service.

Late that evening Noel told me that he wanted to attend the mass. That meant that I would have to stay home to put the children to bed. He planned to pick up his prescription for steroids when he was out and told me in no uncertain terms that I was never to get involved with his MS ever again. He was absolutely mortified at his neurologist's office. He said that he had no idea how far I was willing to take it. I said nothing because I had aggravated him enough and on top of my anger, I felt guilty for upsetting him so much. I promised him that I would never get involved again.

When I put the children to sleep, I logged onto Goodshape's site to update the gang in cyberspace. I told them that I was going to back off all attempts to persuade Noel to try LDN because I felt that I was doing more harm than good. I silently wanted to kill Noel but I didn't share that on the internet. The support from the Goodshape site was instant and sincere. They understood.

Noel arrived home after the memorial mass and to my amazement he was in great spirits with many from the Mom's Group in tow. They all knew the pressure we were under and although I didn't feel like company at the time they are always more than welcome. They had become like family at this stage. I looked at Noel and told him that he had serious nerve to consider me crazy and I asked him whatever happened to the angry guy that left the house earlier. He laughed. He told me that he spent the mass thinking about everything.

He calmed down and like most people at rock bottom, he decided that it was time to pray for guidance. He apologized for implying to his neurologist that I was crazy. Everybody laughed and assured him jokingly that he was probably right. He told me that would try the LDN. He said that if I was that sure about it then maybe Saint Anthony had a hand in it all. He trusted that I had researched it as well as it seemed, and he concluded that maybe it was worth a shot. I told him that it no longer bothered me what he did and I said that he could take LDN or lump it because it was all the same to me.

Tia and Rachel thumped me at that point. Rachel really whacked me on the arm. I laughed at their facial expressions and understood that they were trying to tell me that I got what I wanted after all that time, so I just stopped being angry. Noel gave me the LDN prescription so I could get it filled in the morning. I took it and we called a truce. Noel made a pitcher of margaritas and we all just hung out. It turned into a fun night.

John compounded the LDN and Noel started 3mg LDN September 12th 2002. At the time Noel was also still taking Avonex because he had just received a month's supply. He also started a course of steroids that night, Prednisone, I believe. I told Noel that he had to stop the Avonex for the LDN to work properly because Avonex suppresses the immune system whereas LDN boosts it.

That was incredibly difficult for him to do. His neurologist had told him that although he may have been doing poorly, he would have been a great deal worse off if he hadn't been taking Avonex. Copaxone is the only MS medication that doesn't work by suppressing the immune system so I explained to Noel that he could take the Copaxone with the LDN but said that most of the people reporting success on LDN were taking LDN alone. Noel was very nervous and rightly so. To take LDN, he had to go against what his neurologist thought best for him. I cannot express how difficult that was for him and to be honest I still cannot believe he went for it. I mean really, who would listen to their spouse over their neurologist? Who should?

Noel decided that he would try LDN on its own but if he started to decline really rapidly then he would start the Copaxone immediately. He hated a weekly injection and the thought of one daily was not very appealing. It was a very scary time but we were united and that felt good. Noel stopped the Avonex injections towards the end of September 2002 and replaced them with LDN. He never did start the Copaxone.

In the midst of all of the craziness in August, I called my Aunt Annie to tell her that LDN may hold hope for Neilus and his Parkinsons. I also told Mom that it held tremendous hope for her breast cancer. It amazes me the different ways people react to LDN. With Noel I had to pump LDN and with Neilus I had to deflate it. Neilus was willing to hop on the first plane and meet with Dr. Bihari to see what the guy had to offer. Neilus was so easy to work with in comparison to Noel. I actually kept telling Neilus not to get his hopes up too high but also said that if I was him I would certainly check it out. Neilus instantly wanted to know everything and Annie told me to make an appointment with Dr. Bihari for Neilus. I called Dr. Bihari early September and made an appointment for Neilus for October 4th 2002.

So, just as Noel was starting the LDN, Mom, Dad, Annie and Neilus arrived at the airport. I went to meet them and I immediately noticed that Neilus had progressed. In Irish tradition there was no point telling me or preparing me for the fact that he had progressed. A quick short shock at the airport is considered better than weeks of worry. In keeping with traditions, I told Neilus that he never looked better. At this point I had read far too much about Parkinsons and that night I asked Annie if Neilus was taking any of the standard Parkinsons medications.

As with MS, there is nothing to stop the progression of Parkinsons, but there are medications to control the symptoms. These medications are not without some brutal side effects and I knew that Neilus could hardly tolerate an aspirin let alone the most common medication for Parkinsons, levadopa. Neilus has a hernia and his stomach is very sensitive to medication. I could tell that Annie was worried but she hid it well. We were all worried because it was likely that Neilus would have to suffer Parkinsons without any medication because the chances of him being able to tolerate anything were very slim.

It was so nice to have the gang visit. I needed them and so did Noel. They are amazing people because of their ability to see good in everything. Neilus and Dad checked out our house and quickly started devising a plan to make it better. It needed a paint job and the back yard needed gutting. They were delighted that they would have something to do to pass the time. Mom and Annie promised to make it easy for them to get their work done by taking the kids to the Mall daily. The kids adore their grandparents. Of course they would, it is like Christmas everyday when they are around. Everyone was really happy.

I remember one night when we were going to bed, Noel told me how much he admired my family. He said that he loved them because they really understood life. I knew what he meant. Although he had only been on LDN for about two weeks or so, we had resumed our ability to be intimate again. I don't think that either of us will ever take that for granted in future.

Chapter 17

October 4th came and I was nervous. I was very nervous, but in true Irish style, I completely hid it. To be honest I don't know what I was thinking that day because what we ended up doing made no sense whatsoever. The appointment with Dr. Bihari was at 3:30 p.m.

Dad was eager to paint the whole downstairs of our house that day and started preparing to paint as soon as he woke up. Noel went to work as usual in the morning and I logged on to the internet to print out the directions to Dr. Bihari's office. Although the address seemed to be in a reputable area of New York, I still had no idea what to expect. I was very aware that I had no real knowledge of Dr. Bihari, because I had not actually met him and all references I had regarding his work came from one phone call and cyberspace.

I love Neilus and I really wanted the day to go well. So, being used to doctor appointments that lasted about twenty minutes, I decided that Mom, Annie and the three girls should accompany us. After the consultation I thought we could do something fun in New York together. It seemed to be a reasonable plan at the time. To make sure we arrived on time I suggested we pile into the car at 2:00 p.m.. What a day lay ahead. Dad had his overalls on and paint brush ready on our departure so we waved goodbye to him and we headed for New York. My dad is special. There is nothing he cannot do. He is smart too, because there was no way he was going to join us in New York that day.

I knew my way up until we crossed the George Washington Bridge. As we were crossing I explained to the gang that I needed a navigator. Neilus assumed the position because the grannies in the back could not hear me with the want for a bathroom break among the children. Neilus quickly discovered that he had forgotten his reading glasses so the pair in the back shared theirs. Apparently they all have the same prescription.

I could not hear what he was saying so we got lost. We laughed because we ended up in the slums of New York. We knew that New York is a grid and that it was no big deal because we had the address but time was becoming an issue. We honestly laughed so much that the children kept asking us what was so funny and the more they asked the more we laughed.

We finally found the address with about five minutes to spare. Annie and Neilus decided that I should attend the consultation with Dr. Bihari and Neilus. I was very keen to do so and I figured that they knew that. I really wanted to meet Dr. Bihari and I had many questions. I told the gang to sit tight in the car and I added that we wouldn't be long. We would most likely be half an hour I told them, so we parked in front of the building.

Neilus and I entered 29th West 15th Street. We got into the elevator and on exit we were greeted by Dr. Bihari's wife. She was very friendly. She took Neilus' details and starting telling us that her husband "Bernie" had no idea how to relax. She said that she was concerned for his health because he had no idea how to switch off from his work.

"Dr. Bihari is a workaholic!" she exclaimed.

Neilus can relate well to workaholics because he is the ultimate workaholic himself, because he loves what he does. We both thought that Annie would have been able to relate well to this lady. I only ever met Mrs. Bihari once, but I remember her as a beautiful woman.

Dr. Bihari called us in quite promptly. His office was by no means your typical doctor's office nor was he your typical doctor. I felt like we were entering his living room. Dr. Bihari made us both feel instantly at home. I immediately scanned the area and liked the fact that he had pictures of his family surrounding him. His degrees and certificates, although many and present, were by no means the focus. Dr. Bihari looked to be about seventy, in good health and wore a suit that he was comfortable in. We sat on a very comfortable sofa like piece of furniture and Dr. Bihari looked at Neilus and asked him what he did for a living. I instantly liked Dr. Bihari. It was very apparent from the start that he cared, so I relaxed. I knew that Dr. Bihari asked that question to see if the Parkinsons was related to Neilus' profession but I also knew that if Neilus liked to talk about anything it was his work.

Neilus has a passion for boats. He spent his life building, buying, selling and dealing with boats. He is the type of guy that can wear a suit to convince the politicians to let him run the island ferryboat or a pair of overalls covered in grease to fix an engine. I always enjoy Neilus. He is great with people and it was amusing to listen to him describe his accomplishments so modestly to Dr. Bihari, but he did tell the doctor all that he needed to know.

Neilus travels a great deal, he works twelve hour days and often works the shipyard in Downings, Donegal. Neilus explained that although he was diagnosed with Parkinsons about a year ago he really had it for about three years. He said that it was slowly getting worse. At this stage his arm had a very obvious tremor and his facial expression was pretty blank. Neilus also had a mild tremor in his right leg and his gait was affected because his steps were shorter than average. Dr. Bihari examined Neilus and confirmed that he had Parkinsons. Apparently, Neilus had certain reflexes that were not working right and Dr. Bihari said these made the diagnosis easy. Then Dr. Bihari took a complete health history. I had been to many doctors through Noel but I was impressed with how thorough Dr. Bihari was. I also could not believe how relaxed he was.

The cause of Parkinsons always bothered Neilus because nobody in our family ever had it and we can go back for generations and generations. Dr. Bihari asked him to describe what was going on in his life when he first noticed the symptoms. Neilus explained his personal theory. He said that when the symptoms started it was during one of the most stressful periods of his life and he always wondered if it was the stress that triggered it. Dr. Bihari said that in his experience as a doctor he could not rule out stress as a major factor.

Dr. Bihari explained it like this. He said that we are all born with a particular set of genes that make us genetically susceptible to certain cancers and illnesses from birth. What struck him most in his profession was how common it was for people to contract cancer or some other illness a year or two after retirement in particular. Dr. Bihari said that he thought that after a stressful event, especially as we age, whatever it is that we are genetically predisposed to get, most likely we will get it. He explained that the stress may trigger a susceptible gene, but then it takes time for the symptoms to show. He said that he believes that LDN could prevent many of those illnesses from occurring because many of the illnesses involve the immune system. In his experience, he explained again that everyone with an autoimmune disease has low levels of endorphins and by taking LDN nightly this problem is rectified and the immune system becomes capable of functioning properly and keeps disease at bay. That was why he had taken LDN himself for the last ten years, he told us. He felt that LDN was helping him beat the odds of getting sick.

I asked him what makes the endorphin levels plummet. He said that he didn't know for sure but was convinced that stress and aging were key factors. Dr. Bihari told us that once endorphin levels drop they are not able to come back up on their own. He said that is what LDN is for. I asked him if there was a blood test to determine the exact state of Neilus' endorphins. He explained that there is one but it is not your typical test and it is not that straightforward. He said that he didn't feel that Neilus needed blood work because the testing he did on people in the early days of his discovery confirmed for him that all people with an autoimmune disease have low levels of endorphins. He was pretty sure that Neilus would not turn out to be any different. Dr. Bihari was also pretty sure that Parkinsons is an autoimmune disease.

Everything he said really did make sense. It made sense to a pair in dire need of a way to stop Parkinsons at any rate. Neilus proceeded to ask Dr. Bihari about Parkinsons. Neilus asked him why he thought LDN would work for Parkinsons. Parkinson's Disease is a chronic progressive neurological disease that affects a small area of nerve cells in an area of the brain known as the substantia nigra. These cells normally produce dopamine, a chemical that transmits signals between areas in the brain that, when working normally, coordinate smooth and balanced muscle movement. Parkinson's Disease causes these nerve cells to die, and as a result, body movements are affected. Dr. Bihari believes that in Parkinsons the immune system attacks the substantia nigra. He said that is why he believes it is autoimmune and that was why he figured that LDN would work for Parkinsons. Although it was too early to say for sure how well LDN would work for Parkinsons, Dr. Bihari was convinced at the time that it would stop it progressing. He told Neilus about his three patients with Parkinsons on LDN for a year and who by all accounts were proving his theory.

He was actually telling Neilus that he was pretty sure that Neilus would not progress any further. How unbelievable is that? He said that he would have a clearer view of things in a year or so but reiterated that it looked very promising. It was a great deal of information to take in and believe but we did.

Neilus and I have many similar traits and one of those is our ability to get completely absorbed in something and completely forget about everything else. That day, we completely forgot about the gang in the car. We were nearly two hours into the appointment when we heard a car alarm on the street. I looked at my watch and thought I had better check on them.

I went out to the elevator and stood waiting for it to arrive. My mind was racing. I could hardly take in all I had heard. I realized that if even a fraction of Dr. Bihari's theories were true, then millions of families stood to be helped. I started to make a mental list of questions that I needed to ask him when I had the chance. I then noticed that the elevator was taking a long time to arrive and I realized that I forgot to press the calling button. By the time I got downstairs, the car alarm was off. Looking back, I don't think that it was our car alarm. I opened the front door and I could see the gang in the car laughing, so I headed back upstairs.

I asked Dr. Bihari why he thought the medical community did not recognize the drug. He told me that he had been trying for years to get a clinical trial underway. He said that he desperately wanted a scientific clinical trial of LDN and AIDS. The main problem he said was that LDN is cheap. To get the drug FDA approved for AIDS or MS would cost a couple of million he said, and because the drug is cheap and already FDA approved at the higher dose, nobody in the U.S. would make a profit. He told me that he was more than eager to have his work scrutinized in the hope that LDN would reach the masses and gain scientific recognition. He said that his biggest concern was that he was getting on in years and that he may not be around long enough to see it all through.

I asked him if he tried outside the U.S. He said that he was trying to work with developing countries around the world with a view to LDN and AIDS. He explained that he had initiated a project for the developing world called The Developing Nations Project and that he started a foundation called the Foundation For Immunological Research in an effort to get things off the ground. He shared that he was not having a great deal of luck as of yet but he said that the internet was proving to be the tool that he was waiting for to help get the word out. Dr. Bihari added that he was willing to travel anywhere in the world to conduct a trial if a reputable body was willing to set one up.

It was difficult not to like the guy.

I asked him if he remembered talking with me on the phone a while back. He said that he did and he asked me what my husband decided to do. I told him that Noel had started 3mg LDN after a grueling appointment with his neurologist. I told him about the appointment and Dr. Bihari laughed, and so did I. I told him that Noel's neurologist really thought that I needed therapy. Noel's neurologist was actually looking out for me because he is a decent guy who thought that he was doing the right thing.

I told Dr. Bihari that although Noel was taking LDN, he was not convinced that it would work. I explained that Noel has to play things safe and that he has to mentally prepare for the worst because then if it happens he is ready. Noel, I explained, would never think that LDN would stop his MS because that would make him too vulnerable. He would never leave himself so wide open. I, on the other hand, I explained, had no problem whatsoever believing that LDN would work and should his MS progress again I would deal with it then. For now, his MS was going to stop in my mind.

Dr. Bihari told me to explain to Noel that he should up his dose to 4.5mg because although 3mg works for 85% of people, 4.5mg works for all. The dose is still small so he thought it safer to cover all bases. I asked him about side effects for Neilus and explained my concern that Neilus may not tolerate LDN. Dr. Bihari told me that LDN is very easily tolerated. The most common side effects he said are vivid dreams and some restless nights for a week or two but nothing major. He also assured me that LDN could be safely taken with any other medication except narcotics.

I asked if Neilus or Noel should wear a medical bracelet in case they were in an accident. Dr. Bihari thought not. He said that the dose is so low that it does not stay in the system long enough to be a serious medical threat. If Neilus was in an accident and given narcotics for example, they would not kill him. I told Dr. Bihari that my mom was in the car and he remembered that she had breast cancer. I asked him if I could make an appointment for her before she flew back to Ireland. His wife checked his schedule but there was nothing available. He told me that it was clear to him that she should be on LDN and offered to write her a script. I was delighted. I wanted to put my entire family on it immediately.

When he wrote the script for Neilus and Mom he started on a third. It was for Noel. He gave it to me in case I had trouble getting a renewal from Noel's neurologist. I was so relieved because I was dreading another battle with Noel's neurologist. We thanked Dr. Bihari and we left. We were speechless in the elevator. We felt great. It was a great deal of hope to take in for one day.

We decided to head to Irmat's Pharmacy in NYC to fill the prescriptions right away. Dr. Bihari specifically recommended Irmats. We got to the car and I told the gang that we had to hurry because Irmats closed at six o'clock, which gave us less than ten minutes to find them. The children still needed a bathroom break and the grannies were singing their favorite song for children, "Wheels on the Bus." They looked shattered but happy.

We headed for Irmats. I went in to get the LDN and when I was in Irmats a car alarm went off. This time I assumed that it was somebody else's so I took my time. When I got back to the car I discovered that it was our car alarm and the children were crying. Car alarms and elevators set the children off every time. Neilus was pacing outside the car and the grannies looked numb. I tried to turn off the alarm but I couldn't.

A passerby told us that The Empire State Building was responsible. Car alarms all over the city were going off uncontrollably. As we waited for about an hour and a half for AAA, many complete strangers tried to help us turn it off. I love New York. I have no idea why anyone would think it unfriendly. I love the people. Finally a guy succeeded in switching off the alarm which we just couldn't believe. He lived locally and his name was Jarmane. He was so excited by his accomplishment that he jumped up and punched the air three times. He was a character and we laughed. We thanked him for all his help and headed for home.

I think that all of the passengers were relieved to hit the Jersey side of the George Washington Bridge because it had been a long day. We were all glad to get home. Dad had finished his paint job and the house looked great. He asked the girls if they had fun in New York. They told him that they had the best day ever and they meant it. That made the grannies crack up laughing. I told him that we did have a great day and I really meant it too. We were all so relieved after the consultation with Dr. Bihari that I honestly don't think anything could have dampened our spirits.

Mom has a similar view of her cancer as Noel has of his MS. It is all in God's hands, so whether she took LDN or didn't take LDN, mattered very little to her. However, she knew what I had just experienced with Noel, so she decided to humor me on the basis that it could do her no harm. She refused to cause me any grief whatsoever. That night, October 4th 2002, Neilus, Mom and Noel started 4.5mg LDN nightly.

Chapter 18

I remember feeling delighted that evening. I was filled with hope. I was tired but very happy. Annie asked me what she should expect. I told her that LDN is not a cure. Dr. Bihari's theory is that Neilus would not reach a point lower than his lowest point pre LDN. I told her to think of his worst possible day. I explained that had to be the measuring stick. If he dipped below that point then we would start to question it all, but until then I told her that I was prepared to believe Dr. Bihari. He seemed very compassionate and genuine and he really believed what he said to be true. He was absolutely not a quack or a gangster.

The biggest question in my mind even back then, was exactly how right was Dr. Bihari? I believed the stories in cyberspace and I had no doubt that he had discovered something big, but how big was always the question. I figured that only time would tell, we would just have to wait and see how effective LDN really was.

At first the improvements were stark. Noel really started to pull back very fast. It was incredible. Within six weeks his bladder had greatly improved and he stopped falling over. Although he still needed his cane around the house he was able to take six or seven steps without it. Although there were improvements, the most amazing thing for me was that the onslaught had finally stopped. Noel's MS had stopped progressing. For the first time ever, I think I felt that his MS was under arrest and that was incredibly liberating. As always, Noel remained calm. He didn't get overly excited because mentally he did not buy into it all. Our friends could not believe the visible improvement in him. They were happy days.

Mom, Dad, Annie and Neilus flew back to Ireland early November. Shortly after they left, my younger brother Kevin and his wife Lisa moved in with us because they were attempting a transfer to the U.S..

They stayed with us for about three months before returning to Ireland to settle. Sadly, the U.S. job market was stagnant due to September 11th. Still, it was nice to have the company for a while. Kevin is probably the most reserved member of our family. He is very patient and kind, and thankfully, he too had found his perfect woman. By the time they arrived I think that Noel had reached his plateau. They deduced that he looked the same as he did in Ireland back in May. That was huge to me because I knew that Noel had slipped a great deal between May and September. For a while MS went into the background and once again, life took over.

I kept in constant contact with Neilus and Annie. We discarded tradition and agreed that our communication would always be open and honest. As time passed it became obvious that Neilus' Parkinsons had also stopped progressing. He told me that he was doing better than ever. He was even able to weld again. Honestly, it was incredible.

Mom was more difficult to measure. She felt the same on LDN as she did before she started it. She didn't notice any difference. I felt relieved that she was taking LDN and I stopped worrying before her routine checkups.

All in all, things were great. Noel, Mom and Neilus were healthy again and thriving thanks to Dr. Bihari and LDN. Life was very good and was to remain so for quite some time. Thank God, we were given a break at last. It was a pleasure to ring in 2003.

It is odd, as I try to write the next part of this story that I should find it so difficult. It is now January 2005 and much has happened since January 2003. Before I continue, I will share that word has leaked out among friends and family regarding my ambition to give a true account of my experiences with LDN and the reception is mixed. I suppose the bottom line is that my nearest and dearest as always are naturally trying to protect me. I fear that some feel that I am fighting a useless fight. I really and truly don't think so. My ambition with regard to this story is clear in my mind. I want to give a true account as to how Parkinsons, breast cancer, and in particular MS have affected my life and how I believe that there is tremendous hope for all people in a boat similar to mine.

I want to see a scientific trial for a cheap drug that holds great promise for millions. I don't expect or want anybody to take my word that the drug works. Instead, I want to see pressure put on a government to take the initiative. The Irish Government is a reasonable target because they stand to gain much financially. As the story unfolds it will become clear that I am not alone in this quest, far from it. Many who have also seen or experienced first hand the implications of this medication also feel a moral obligation to share. That will become very clear. But before I continue, it is also important that I share one more thing.

I have to date, received many e-mails of gratitude from people all around the world who have started LDN and have experienced much benefit. When I read of references referring to my altruistic nature, it is important that I clarify. As I have written, I have three children. Since becoming a mother I relate much better to my own mother. My every breath is for them. In my mind they are possibly genetically predisposed to acquire an autoimmune disorder. Should that be so, I want to challenge Dr. Bihari's theory because if he is right, the outcome of a trial would certainly shed a great deal more light on how to treat a variety of such disorders.

Today, most people with an autoimmune disorder, are basically given steroids and antibiotics. There is no treatment, just symptom management. An LDN trial could potentially redirect future research and improve millions of lives. Although I deeply feel for and empathize with all families afflicted with illness, I also fear for my children. I am not certain what drives me most, but I believe that it is a combination of motherhood and moral duty. It basically comes down to a feeling that regardless of how the last page writes, this is the right thing to do. It is a story that I strongly feel has to be shared. What if Dr. Bihari is right? That is the ultimate bottom line.

The promise LDN holds outweighs by far any personal embarrassment on my part. To find the truth I am more than willing to put myself out there and suffer the consequences. To start with I want to see a scientific clinical trial for LDN and MS. MS, because that is where the overwhelming testimonies lie. From there, who knows? So, I will continue, starting back at January 2003.

As January 2003 passed I became more and more convinced that LDN was working. Noel was without question stable. He no longer had to heave himself off the couch and for the first time in about ten years his feet were warm again. His complexion was also much better. I remember thinking that he just looked healthy. The biggest benefit was of course that the onslaught had stopped. Noel's spirits were as always good.

We didn't discuss LDN much at the time. Just as Noel never wanted to make MS his life, I knew that he would not want to make LDN his life either. He wanted to get on with life as best he could and so did I. I really think that I actually forgot about MS for a while. I stopped reading the Goodshape message board and I rarely researched anything on the internet. Life was very good.

I decided to take another trip back to Ireland in February 2003. The girls and I traveled ahead of Noel and as always he joined us for the second two weeks. This time he brought his own wheelchair and his journey went without incident. I really enjoyed that visit. It was the first time that we were without Noel and I was not worried about him having a relapse when we were gone. I believed that the LDN would hold him and it did.

People in Ireland who had not seen Noel since May 2002 thought that he looked the same. That was a great testimony for LDN in my book because they missed his rapid decline. Also, it felt good to see Neilus thriving again. Like Noel, he looked healthy. To me his shake was less visible. Unlike Noel, Neilus was very open about how good he felt on LDN initially. He was openly in shock that the drug was proving to be effective. Like Noel, Neilus insisted on taking one day at a time. They both agreed, that as with MS, the course in Parkinsons is unknown, but they acknowledged that it looked very promising. For Noel to think LDN promising, was a huge step forward in my mind.

Chapter 19

When we had settled back into New Jersey that spring, my close friend from the Mom's Group with MS, started to slip. She was using the same neurologist as Noel. I consider this lady one of my closest friends and I desperately wanted her to take LDN because I believed that it was working wonders for Noel. I thought that seeing as she had witnessed the effect LDN had on Noel, she would just start to take it without question. It was not that straight forward.

I had to convince her as I did Noel and she proved to be just as stubborn with less reason in my mind. For a start, she refused all MS medications anyway so she didn't have to stop any drug in order to take it. Also, she had visible proof that it was working, not just stories from cyberspace. And, I assured her that Dr. Bihari was legitimate and genuine. I could not believe her resistance, but I would never judge or question it because I have no idea what it is actually like to have MS. I may have reacted exactly the same way myself.

She told me that the fact she had already refused MS medications automatically made her less likely to consider LDN. I never understood that, but I don't have to.

My friend's MS was invisible but affecting her life. She was very tired every evening and her legs would just give in sometimes when she climbed the stairs. Often, she was not able to climb the stairs when the day ended. Her legs were numb and tingling but all of her symptoms always came and went. She has relapsing remitting MS and steroids always set her straight. She was not too keen on the LDN idea but she decided to discuss it with Noel.

Noel told her that if he were her, he would try it just because it wouldn't do her any harm. He said that it helped him a bit, but he didn't think that it helped him as much as everybody else said and claimed to see it did. He said that he still had no feeling in his legs but he was glad that at least he looked good to others. He could not have played it down more. My friend remained hesitant.

She went to see her neurologist and he told her that he had one patient on LDN but that as far as he knew it had no effect. He told her that he discussed LDN with his colleagues and they decided it best not to prescribe it in future. Noel had not been back to see the neurologist at this stage so the neurologist assumed that LDN had failed Noel. My friend was aware of my meeting with her neurologist so she decided it best not to acknowledge that she knew me.

My friend asked her neurologist if he would write her a prescription for LDN. She said that she had decided that she would like to try it. Her neurologist refused to write her a prescription for LDN and he told her that she should really consider the shots. She refused and left his office with a blast of steroids.

A couple of weeks passed and I remember calling round to my friend's house. Her symptoms were still bothering her. I told her that it was time that she met with Dr. Bihari. She was still on the fence but I put the phone in her hand and told her to make an appointment, because enough was enough. She called and made an appointment. Her husband and her met Dr. Bihari on March 8th 2003. Everybody I know who has met with Dr. Bihari has a story and I laughed out loud when I heard theirs.

My friend said that she was taken back when she first met Dr. Bihari. He was just after a hip operation and he needed a cane to get around. She thought that he looked like death and she could not believe that I didn't prepare her for the shock. I laughed because when I met him in October he looked like a healthy seventy year old to me. Although he had been on LDN for ten years, I would agree that he wasn't exactly a poster child for it, but still he was healthy. I also laughed when I thought of what his wife must have been saying to him because I knew that his workaholic tendency bothered her. I just pictured her begging him to at least rest after surgery. I respected and liked Dr. Bihari even more for working immediately after surgery. It showed his dedication and belief in what he was doing. My friend and her husband quickly settled, and I think they also felt his compassion.

My friend started LDN mid March 2003. She started with the same mind set as Noel. She did not believe that her MS would not progress. It was simply too dangerous for her to think like that. She figured that based on the fact that LDN had no side effects and was cheap, she would try it. Also, her insurance covered her consult with Dr. Bihari so everything worked in her favor.

Initially she felt wonderful on LDN. She could not believe how great she felt and I was so happy for her. She had a great deal more energy and she could not wait to tell her neurologist her success story. But then the unthinkable happened.

In July 2003 my friend started to relapse on LDN. I did not understand how was that possible, because at that time I had never heard of anybody relapse on LDN. All of her old symptoms came back with a vengeance. She did not experience anything brand new, but her symptoms became more severe than she ever remembered. I even remember noticing that she developed foot drop, and her ability to stand for any period of time had greatly diminished. That was a very scary time.

My friend seemed to be proving that the LDN theory was not true and she was ready to pack it in. One day during her relapse she called to my house and she phoned Dr. Bihari to tell him what was happening to her. He told her to eat three bars of chocolate a day for the next three days. She hung up and we looked at each other in disbelief and for the first time ever, I began to wonder if Dr. Bihari was a quack because his advice sounded crazy. I decided that I had to investigate thoroughly.

My mind initially went back to the consult with Neilus and my gut still believed him. I had already thoroughly checked out his credentials and I judged his character to be honest. Growing up in the hotel business I like to think gives me an edge in this field. Whether or not I had to believe in Dr. Bihari for sanity I don't know, but I do know that I was not prepared to give up on LDN so easily.

I remembered that Dr. Bihari said that LDN would only reverse the last three months of MS scarring on the spinal cord or brain for the lucky people and that all old scars would remain. Also, I remembered that he said that in times of personal stress or infection (fever, flu, etc) the old scars may flare up causing a reoccurrence of old symptoms, but he firmly believed that no new symptoms would develop. My friend did not experience any brand new symptoms so I began to think that maybe the theory was still true. She didn't seem stressed though and she didn't look like she was running an infection, but something was clearly not right. It wasn't clear what was causing her olds scars to flare up.

I logged on to the Goodshape site and started to investigate. I posted two questions. I asked if any of them were aware of anybody who had relapsed while on LDN and I explained my friend's situation. Then I asked, what the connection was, between chocolate and LDN. The replies were most helpful and explained a great deal.

They told me that it was quite common for old symptoms to return in full force shortly after starting LDN. Some considered this a good sign and referred to it as a healing crisis. My friend didn't really fall into this category because initially she was doing better than ever. She seemed to start to slip out of the blue after initial improvement so it could not have been a healing crisis.

Then a woman named Angelina spotted the problem. She convinced me that my friend was probably suffering from invisible candida, a simple yeast infection, as a result of her steroid use pre LDN. Angelina had suffered similar infections and to her knowledge the LDN would be more effective if this problem was addressed. She then told me about a simple test that my friend could perform to confirm whether or not her yeast levels were too high. My friend really thought that if she was running a yeast infection that she would know about it, but to humor me she took the test. I was happy when the test revealed that her yeast levels were very high.

A couple of days later, her mouth broke out in sores. My friend, without question had a yeast infection. She addressed this infection, but had lost confidence in LDN. She was not convinced that something so simple would set off all of her symptoms. She was also planning a trip to Disney with her family so she called her neurologist and began a course of steroids to get by. That was July 2003. My friend did not stop taking LDN, she continued to take it and all of her symptoms slowly disappeared again.

My friend has not taken steroids since then, but she assures me that she will relapse any day now and need them. That initial setback, understandably, left her more than cautious. I think that she is doing wonderful, but like everyone on LDN, when she is stressed or running an infection her old symptoms do flare up. Thank God, she has not experienced any brand new symptoms. Her MS has not progressed. Although she does not believe in LDN, she will not stop taking it, but she insists that she remains mentally prepared for progression and more relapses.

The Goodshape board also educated me on the connection between chocolate and LDN. Many told me that they found it beneficial during times of stress. Even my friend said at the time that she felt a bit better taking it. It turns out that there is an amino acid called DL Phenylalanine in chocolate, and it slows the breakdown of endorphins during the day. Dr. Bihari believes that this works well with LDN because it helps to keep endorphin levels higher for longer daily. Many on the board had chocolate allergies so knew to take the capsule supplement from any vitamin store instead. Some said that it worked wonders, and others said that it didn't.

I have since spoken to Dr. Bihari about this and he now recommends the supplement instead of chocolate. He recommends 500mg DL Phenylalanine in the morning and afternoon in times of stress or infection to help boost the LDN effect.

Noel, Neilus and my close friend completely convinced me that Dr. Bihari really had discovered something big. Although they could not mentally buy into it all, watching them was proof enough for me.

At this stage, April 2004, Noel had been taking LDN for about nine months with no progression. He went to see his neurologist but I didn't go. I don't specifically remember being invited. After the neurological exam it was decided that Noel was the same as before and his neurologist advised him to just keep on doing whatever he was doing.

My friend has since been to see the same neurologist and tried to convince him that she really thinks that there is something in LDN, but he assured her that there isn't. He told her that if she remains relapse free for about three years then maybe he would start to look into it. He still feels that she should take the shots.

Their neurologist is an excellent neurologist by the way. I believe that he is quite a typical neurologist.

Chapter 20

One day in the middle of the summer in 2003, I decided that it was time to let people know about LDN. I really wanted every family to benefit as mine had done. I hated to think of all the people progressing with MS, Parkinsons or any autoimmune disorder when there is something so simple available to help them all.

Since that time I have met many people who have truly amazed and inspired me. I have also learned much as to how the world works. It has been an interesting journey to say the least.

Ireland seemed like the most sensible place to start in my mind because the Irish Government pays for all of the costly MS medications there. I began to investigate how many people in Ireland were taking LDN. I was already aware of one lady I spoke with on the Goodshape message board back in September 2002. Her name was Mauka.

During that period in 2002 when Noel's job was insecure, I was trying to figure out how he would obtain LDN if we had to move back to Ireland. This was before I met Dr. Bihari and discovered that Irmats Pharmacy ship worldwide. Anyway, Mauka was incredibly helpful.

She heard about LDN through the Goodshape site and she was based in Wicklow. Her neurologist is based in St. Vincent's in Dublin. She told me that her neurologist was more than skeptical about prescribing LDN and it took a great deal of convincing on her part to actually get the prescription. On top of that, she then had to find somewhere in Ireland to make up the LDN.

In the States, a compounding pharmacy generally takes the FDA approved 50mg naltrexone tablets, pulverizes them, and compounds 4.5mg LDN capsules. The most important requirement when compounding LDN is that the filler used in the capsule ensures the fast release of the drug into the body. Although the expertise is available in Ireland to do this, the technology to make 4.5mg LDN capsules is not. However, liquid LDN also ensures fast release and liquid LDN was starting to take off in the States at the time. People who were finding it difficult to get a prescription from their neurologist were legally importing 50mg naltrexone tablets from Mexico, with the brand name Revia. They would then split a pill in half, pulverize it and add 25ml of water, shake it, let it dissolve and drink 4.5ml nightly. Most people crushed half a pill at a time to ensure freshness. People on liquid LDN were reporting great success. Many preferred this for a number of reasons. It ruled out compounding errors, it was even cheaper than the capsules and they could adjust their dose very easily until they found what worked best for them. Some did not like this method because a 50mg naltrexone pill weighs about 315mg, meaning that it contains a filler and this filler is not soluble, so the homemade liquid shot of LDN is a little lumpy.

In Ireland, a pharmacy on Lower Lesson Street in Dublin, had a pharmacist named Ann, and she made up the LDN prescription for Mauka in a solution that stayed fresh for two weeks. Mauka received her LDN by post every two weeks in Wicklow from Dublin. Also, the Health Board for the Wicklow area covered the cost of Mauka's LDN under the Long Term Illness program. Mauka was delighted to be on LDN. Like everyone else with whom I was in contact at the time, she was stable. My last contact with her was in October 2003. She had just gone for her annual appointment with her neurologist and he detected no deterioration in her condition for the year she was on LDN. But better than that, she felt great within herself. She knew that she had not progressed and she had no desire to ever stop taking LDN. As far as I know, Mauka was the first person in Ireland to take LDN. In July 2003 she was the only person, besides Mom and Neilus, I could find in Ireland on LDN.

Chapter 21

I searched around a bit more to try to find out if there were others in Ireland taking LDN and when I could not find any, I decided to check out Britain. I came across a doctor in Wales name Dr. Robert Lawrence. He was easy to find because he has his own website with all of his information. He has MS himself and he started taking LDN after reading about Dr. Bihari's work on Goodshape's site. He was so impressed with the results that he started to prescribe LDN for MS patients. He altered Dr. Bihari's theory slightly.

Dr. Lawrence does not recommend taking LDN every night in case the body becomes dependant or develops a tolerance. He recommends that people come off LDN for two days after every ten days on the drug. Most people seem to adhere to Dr. Bihari's method however, and take LDN every night because he is the founding father of it all and he is convinced that there is no need for intermittent therapy because of the low dose required. Also, LDN is used more widely in the U.S. where many people have never heard of Dr. Lawrence's concerns, so they just follow Dr. Bihari.

At this stage in July 2003, I believe that Dr. Lawrence was importing LDN from the States, but in time Martindale Pharmaceuticals in the U.K. started to supply him. The LDN movement was much more advanced in Britain than in Ireland thanks to the efforts of Dr. Lawrence. As in the States, people with MS all over Britain were reporting wonderful success stories on LDN on the internet. What was most remarkable was that LDN did seem to work for everyone. LDN was working across the board.

It was then that I decided I wanted LDN to really hit Ireland, so I started with the people I knew. Although I had informed Dr. Muriel and Coirle's sister back in August 2002, that I was looking into LDN,

I thought that it was time to update them. I think that like most people they figured that if there was any real truth in what I was saying then their neurologist would know about it.

I remember phoning Dr. Muriel. I will always be grateful to her for the hope she gave me in back in 1998 when I was at my lowest point. I explained the whole LDN theory to her and explained how well it was working for Noel. She told me that she would investigate and asked me to inform the top neurologist in Dublin. I knew that she was referring to Mauka's neurologist. I told her that he was already aware of it and that he even had one patient taking LDN, but she had to fight for her prescription.

I suppose the years have made Dr. Muriel skeptical of miracle treatments for MS, and I certainly do not blame her. Although delighted that LDN was working for Noel, she decided in the end that she would stick with conventional thinking. She told me that the shots were helping her overall. I completely respected her decision and felt good that at least she is now aware of something else should she need it in the future.

I then phoned the sister of my childhood friend Coirle. Her husband Robert, was doing quite poorly at the time. On top of MS he was also starting a battle with another autoimmune illness, sarcoidosis. He was taking a weekly shot of Avonex but they did not feel that it was helping him. I told Coirle's sister all about LDN. I told her that I knew that it sounded too good to be true, but that she had to convince Robert of its merits if he was to have any chance of winning the fight. I also told her that most likely the LDN would also help his sarcoidosis. I explained how difficult it was for me to convince Noel, but that it was worth it in my book. Coirle's sister was very grateful for the information and assured me that she would pass it all on to her husband and told me that she felt very confident that Robert would thoroughly investigate.

At this point in his life, Robert was very tired in the evenings and he could never get enough sleep. He just never felt well rested and he suffered serious joint pain. At times he also used a cane for support. His quality of life was greatly impaired which also affected his wife and their two young children. Robert was on quite a few medications at the time to deal with his symptoms. Coirle's sister told Robert all about LDN and Robert really ran with it. As she predicted, he investigated everything on the internet.

Early July 2003, Robert went to see his neurologist in Galway. His neurologist could see that the Avonex did not seem to be doing Robert any favors and he suggested that Robert discontinued the shots. Robert told him that he was thinking of trying LDN. Robert's neurologist was, quite rightly, political in his reply. He pointed out that there were no formal trials to back up anecdotal testimonies on the internet and that as far as he knew, LDN was not available in Ireland. Robert said that that Dr. Lawrence in Wales could supply him.

The neurologist basically told Robert that if he wanted to go for it to do so, he was not going to try to stop him. He remained very neutral which could be perceived as somewhat supportive. Robert spoke with Dr. Lawrence on the phone very shortly after that and then he sent Dr. Lawrence his medical notes. Robert started 3.5mg LDN nightly mid July 2003 and then he moved up to 4mg towards the end of July.

Robert and his wife could not believe the effect LDN had on him. It was life changing. They thought it nothing short of a miracle. The first thing Robert noticed was that his joint pain disappeared. Then his energy levels soared and his over all general well-being greatly improved. He no longer needed a selection of medications or a cane at all. LDN seemed to cover all the bases. It was unbelievable.

Robert could not believe that the world didn't know about this tiny simple pill. He felt a strong moral obligation to let as many people as possible know about it so he immediately started to spread the word. Robert has since been interviewed many times but I like the story about his trip to Valentia in County Kerry, because it is tangible and powerful testimony for LDN.

A month before Robert started on LDN he went on a business trip to Carlow. A work colleague drove him there and back, but it still took Robert three days to recover from the trip. Then, about a month after going on LDN, he had a business meeting to attend in Valentia, County Kerry. He drove the five hour trip himself, attended a four hour meeting and drove back that same day himself. The following morning he went to work feeling fine. There was no recovery period required.

Then, shortly after that, his LDN supply got stuck in the post. He had to go seven days without it. Within those seven days his fatigue returned and he started to need his stick again. Once he resumed the LDN, the symptoms disappeared as before.

It is important to point out that it was a difficult decision for Robert to come off the Avonex and go on LDN. As with Noel, it was a personal risk that he decided to take. It is a risk that thousands of people have taken because they feel the standard MS medications do not work for them.

The more I talked with people during the summer of 2003 it became clear that LDN needed a scientific clinical trial, so that people would not feel that they were gambling with their lives. I really wanted the fear removed from taking a chance on LDN. At the time I didn't know how to approach the whole issue of a trial, but I knew that the first stage had to be getting the word out.

I figured the best place to start was with the MS Societies. I thought that once they heard about LDN, they would do everything in their power to get scientific recognition for LDN, and help get it to the people who really needed it. There are many people with MS who take no medications at all, people who just refuse the shots, but might consider LDN if they knew about it. I felt that they had a right to know about LDN, and at least make up their own mind as to whether or not they wanted to try it. It was frustrating to feel that I knew something that everybody else should know.

I notice that the MS Ireland website has been changed since summer 2003. Anyway, they still have a letters section to which I wrote a letter about Noel and LDN. I made it clear that the drug needed a scientific trial but that it held tremendous hope, was cheap and had no side effects. I checked the letters page of the website the following morning to see if I could view it but it was not there. So, I wrote the letter again but it never appeared on the website. I tried once more and when it never showed I figured that I was being blocked. MS Ireland did not want me to tell the LDN story and that annoyed me.

I decided to investigate a bit more. I noticed that it is the policy of MS Ireland not to give advice on therapies that are not clinically proven. I respected that, but this was a letters page. This was me telling my story, not MS Ireland pumping LDN. I was simply telling a story in the hope that people could investigate and make up their own minds.

I read some of the other letters. Some spoke of bee stings and others mentioned a particular diet. These were not clinically proven, but yet were opinions that MS Ireland deemed okay to share. I appreciated reading the experience of people on bee stings and diets, but it made me angry that I was not allowed to talk about LDN. I decided to dig deeper.

Then I learned that MS Ireland is pretty much, completely, financially dependant on the drug companies pumping out the expensive MS medications. How wrong is that? If the drug companies want to help people with MS then it should be made very clear, almost in the naming of the societies they sponsor, where the financial interests of such societies rest. For example, why not call MS Ireland, Biogen's MS Ireland if it is true that they have indirect control. That way people could directly applaud Biogen for all the good work that they possibly do to help people with MS. It would also avoid any potential confusion regarding possible conflict of interest when discussing other drugs like LDN for MS. MS Ireland weren't going out of their way to sabotage LDN, they just didn't want to know anything about LDN, or let anyone else know anything about it through them.

I was familiar with some people from various MS societies around Ireland and I knew that these people were good people. I knew that their hearts genuinely lay in the best interests of people with MS, despite the politics of the society. I also knew that many worked for the society because they were directly affected by MS, either they actually had the disease or a loved one did. MS is personal to them so I knew that many would listen. I often wonder how much more some neurologists would listen to the LDN theory if MS was personal to them. I would never wish MS to be personal for anybody but I know that it makes all the difference in the world.

At that time the MS Ireland website had a list of every single MS branch in Ireland, not just the regional head offices, it listed every small branch in every nook and cranny of the country, 39 in total. They even listed the names and phone numbers of the chairperson and secretary of each branch. Also, they had profiles of people with MS living in Ireland complete with their e-mail address. They certainly supplied me with a gold mine of information.

One afternoon that summer, when the children were resting, I started at the top of the phone list. My first phone call was to the Athlone branch and I wasn't nervous at all. I spoke with Eileen. Every phone call I made turned into a lengthy one because not one office had ever even heard of LDN. I averaged about a call or two a day for the next while. It amazed me how quick the people were to share their personal MS nightmares. Eileen told me that she had a mild form of MS and that she considered herself very lucky. In the Ballina Branch, Mary has MS and she is in wheelchair, in Bandon, Padraic's wife has MS for fifteen years, in Bray, Helen's husband is in a wheelchair, in Sligo, Kathleen's husband is bedridden with MS, in Letterkenny, John is battling MS and in Galway, Aidan has a loved one who is also suffering. The list went on and on. It was harrowing. I cannot express how wonderful every representative from each branch was. Many were inspirational in how they dealt with MS or cared for a loved one. They were so passionate, and I could really relate. Many apologized on behalf of MS Ireland that my letter was blocked. They said that they were saddened and shocked. Some took my e-mail address and phone number and promised that they would start to distribute it to the public.

Shortly after my phone calls, I started getting quite a bit of e-mail inquiring about LDN. I replied to most if not all. I also personally e-mailed seventy-two people in Ireland who had their e-mail address openly available on the MS Ireland website. I was busy, but driven. Word about LDN was getting out all around Ireland and it was exciting. People were listening, they were really listening.

Many went straight to Dr. Lawrence in Wales and started LDN almost immediately and reported back tales of success and sincere gratitude. Many of the e-mails contained passionate stories that made a lump form in my throat. It was incredible. I particularly remember a young guy from Galway named Fergal who wanted in the worst way to buy me a drink because he was going to climb Craogh Patrick since he started LDN. There were also others who were hesitant and fearful and chose not to try LDN but still appreciated the knowledge. I didn't receive any negative feedback. It was all very positive. I got to know a great deal of people that summer whom I will never forget. I am sure I will meet many face to face during future trips to Ireland. The best thing about all of it was that as people read about LDN and tried it, they also felt obligated to tell others. It was the snowball effect in essence.

By October 2003, LDN hit the Sunday Post thanks to Robert. This is the article that they printed. LDN was hitting the mainstream media and I, like many others at this stage, felt it imperative to push for a trial.

MS experimental drug could save state millions of euro'
05/10/03 00:00
By Simon Carswell
A handful of multiple sclerosis (MS) sufferers in Ireland have switched to a new medication that costs just 4 per cent of the price of the drug commonly used to treat the disease.

Most of the 6,000 MS patients in the state use a drug called Beta Interferon. However, about a dozen Irish MS sufferers have switched to a drug called Low Dose Naltrexone (LDN), which boosts the immune system and is used to treat HIV/Aids and cancer. A year's supply of Beta Interferon for an MS sufferer costs the state about 12,000, compared to 480 a year for LDN. Most Irish patients buy LDN from Dr. Robert Lawrence, a GP based in Wales who is himself an MS sufferer.

Dr. Lawrence said he has supplied the drug to about a dozen patients in Ireland, mostly in the west. The drug is approved by the FDA in the U.S., but no clinical trials have been carried out on it in Ireland or Britain. He said he explains this to patients before selling them the drug. "I explain when I introduce it to people that what they are using is experimental and that no trials have been carried out on it and that people must accept it as such," said Lawrence.

One MS sufferer, a businessman from Co Galway, said he switched from Beta Interferon to LDN in early August and since then has experienced "a dramatic difference" in health.

"It got rid of my fatigue and my joint pain, and also re-moved weakness in my lower limbs," he said. "I can now work a full day and enjoy more time with my children, and life in general."

He urged the Department of Health to fund clinical trials and research of LDN, as it could save the state millions of euro every year. Lawrence said he imports LDN from New York for resale in Britain and Ireland.

"The only reason I can imagine why no further research or investigation has been done is that, because the drug is so relatively cheap, no drug company is interested in producing it or supporting the trials that will get it accepted as an approved treatment for MS. There is simply no potential for significant profit," he said.

Maura McKeon, spokeswoman for the Multiple Sclerosis Society of Ireland, said: "Until trials are carried out on it, we cannot advise people to try this particular product. Up to now, we have received only anecdotal evidence of its effects."

I felt that things were really happening and that felt good. I was delighted that Noel was still doing great, as was Neilus, my friend from the Mom's Group, Robert and Goodshape's wife, Polly. The LDN website was expanding rapidly and even started its own message board where people gathered to share their personal LDN experience and encourage each other. Other message boards dedicated to LDN also started to appear on the internet. The word was spreading like wildfire. I remember reading the following in October 2003 on the LDN site:

From: Dr. Skip [Skip's Pharmacy, Boca Raton, FL]Re: Naltrexone
Date: Thu Oct 23 18:21:35 2003

As I have said before, if I had MS, the only Drug that I would absolutely be taking is LDN. I wouldn't care what it took, or who I had to insult. In 4 years of dispensing LDN, with over 10,000 patient months, I have heard of only three cases of exacerbation. I am waiting for our new resident to come in and I will have exact numbers, but this is truly a no-brainer. I would find some one to prescribe it no matter the cost or effort.
Dr. Skip

In the midst of all of this, in September 2003 my eldest daughter Annie, started school in New Jersey. I met her teacher, Rosemary Konde, and it is a meeting I will share because it had a deep and probably ever lasting effect on me.

Chapter 22

I had heard of people who met people whom they thought they knew before. I had heard of people who believed that everyone on earth was somebody's angel. I had heard of people who swore that they saw stuff in people nobody else could see. I enjoyed such stories, many of which emanated from my maternal grandmother, but never believed a word. Then I met Rosemary. I think that if I was told that I had an hour left to live I would include her in my thoughts. I wish everyone would meet a Rosemary.

She was in a huge, tastefully and colorfully decorated classroom with her class of awkward five year olds on the floor around her. She sat on a rocking chair and sported a pair of eyeglasses on the tip of her nose. From a distance I estimated that she was sixty or so, but up close she was obviously only in her very early fifties. She had such a pleasant countenance and eyes that just looked at things right.

Like all of the other moms of her class, I believed that Annie could not have landed a better kindergarten teacher and that was important to me, but beyond that, I felt an instant connection with Rosemary before I even spoke with her. I didn't acknowledge the connection but I did sign up to help out with class parties, and I made a note of Rosemary's e-mail address to coordinate such events.

I shared my affections with Tia and we agreed it best that I kept my distance, to let the woman get on with her job. To tell her that she was remarkable, apart from making strained conversation, just sounded so lame that we laughed about it. Often when I would visit Tia, she would ask how "Rosie" was doing and I would show her Annie's schoolwork and tease her that she was wasting her money sending her child to private school. It was all good fun.

Then, around Thanksgiving, which is late November, I e-mailed all of my contacts in Ireland to inform them that I had written to Pat Kenny, a popular talk show host in Ireland. I was eager to get Dr. Bihari on Irish TV and I was convinced that Pat Kenny would jump at the opportunity. I called Dr. Bihari before I sent the letter and I was amazed that he was willing to travel to Ireland to get the word out. As soon as I sent the e-mail I noticed that I included Rosemary by accident. I couldn't believe it. The last thing in the world I wanted was to divulge my LDN obsession with "Rosie."

Like every year, Tia and I met at 5:00 a.m. on the Friday after Thanksgiving to shop in the sales. We get all of our Christmas gifts in one day. That Friday morning, when we were standing in line outside Toys R Us, I told Tia of my e-mail error. Tia laughed so hard because it was funny. We both laughed.

We were also laughing at the time because we just figured out why we were first in line. The store didn't open until 7:00 a.m.. We couldn't believe how wrong we got the time and how many others were there on purpose. The TV crews were setting up and we laughed at the thought of the Mom's Group seeing us in line so early on TV. As a group of young moms we are unique because one of us is always in the midst of some calamity.

Anyway, that Thanksgiving I asked Tia what I should do about "Rosie" and we were torn as to whether or not I should pretend I didn't notice my error or own up to it.

I decided to explain the LDN story to Rosemary in a follow up e-mail. I explained that I feared a plea for sanity would only confirm madness as I understood that the story was difficult for many to believe in the absence of a proper clinical trial. I clearly realized that some people thought that I had to believe in LDN because I could not face the reality of MS. I knew that was not the case.

Rosemary replied to my second e-mail and her reply floored me. If you believe in coincidence, it was a classic. As I mentioned earlier, I don't believe in coincidence. I like to think that everything happens for a reason.

Rosemary explained that a line from my e-mail that struck her was that Dr. Bihari claimed that all autoimmune diseases would respond to LDN. She said that she was absent from school that Wednesday because she was at the hospital with her twenty-six-year-old daughter Kate who needed her third surgery for nasal polyps and deviated septum. She explained that Kate is what is known as a Samters Triad patient, a condition which causes the patient to suffer from asthma, an intolerance to aspirin and severe nasal polyps. She described Kate as having no energy with a perpetual cold and no sense of smell and hence appetite. Then, she said that she believed that Samters is an autoimmune disease.

Rosemary believed that in Samters, the immune system attacks the nasal passages. She had already spent hours on the websites reading about Dr. Bihari and LDN in the hope that it would be helpful to Kate and she planned to bring it all to Kate's attention as soon as possible. By all accounts, Rosemary was delighted to have received the information. She was very glad of my mistake.

Rosemary presented the information to Kate and like her mom, Kate cut to the chase and could see that LDN could potentially help her. I instantly liked Kate. She is a fighter with great spirit and wit. I think that Kate and Rosemary kept their expectations realistic and thought LDN worth a try seeing as it had no side effects. Kate realized that she had little to lose and much to possibly gain by trying it. She took all of the information to her ENT (ear, nose and throat) doctor early December 2003 and as expected he had never heard of LDN and did not want to prescribe it.

Kate immediately called Dr. Bihari. To her amazement, he spoke with her for about twenty-five minutes on the phone and she made an appointment to see him on Friday, December 12th. Her mom, dad, and husband attended the consult with her. I remember that I could not wait to hear how her appointment went and I eagerly awaited the report. It was a good one.

Kate and her family were very impressed with Dr. Bihari. They thought him humble considering his accomplishments. Their appointment lasted about two hours. He said that he had not seen a case like Kate's in thirty years and that her type of immune disease is very rare. He pointed out that in addition to the big and famous immune diseases such as MS and ALS, he believed that there are hundreds of other rare diseases, such as Samters that get very little interest by the medical community because of their low rate of incidence in the population. Dr. Bihari questioned Kate very thoroughly as to her medical history, asthma, allergies, polyps, surgeries and medications. Then, he did a thorough questioning about her family's medical history. He was interested to hear about the juvenile diabetes, sensitivities to red wine and the asthma of her other cousins. He concluded that Kate does indeed have an autoimmune illness and even went so far as to guess that she is also a chronic fatigue patient probably triggered by the mononucleosis she had when she was sixteen. He wanted Kate to start on LDN immediately and after four weeks he wanted to have blood work done to see if the Epstein-Barr virus was still in her system.

Dr. Bihari hoped that Kate's energy levels would increase on the LDN and that no additional medications would be needed, but should she not improve he mentioned an additional prescription that she might need. Kate was amazed that he was able to pinpoint some symptoms that she had forgotten to tell him about, particularly difficulty with short term memory and occasional flare ups of hives for no apparent reason.

Kate felt that Dr. Bihari was one of the first doctors who ever listened to her.

Dr. Bihari also recommended that Rosemary take the LDN as a preventative measure considering six out of nine siblings on her dad's side died of cancer.

They left his office filled with hope. Kate started LDN on Monday December 15th 2003. I was so happy for her and really hoped that she would live happily ever after. I still hope that Kate lives happily ever after.

Christmas 2003 was a wonderful Christmas, probably one of my best. Mom, Dad, Annie and Neilus came to visit us again and Neilus had a follow up appointment with Dr. Bihari on December 17th. When I went to JFK airport to pick them up I immediately noticed how well Neilus looked. He looked great but I couldn't put my finger on it as to why. His shake was still visible, but it was definitely less visible than the previous year.

For this consultation, Neilus and I headed into New York on our own. Dr. Bihari's secretary Bill greeted us when we came out of the elevator on that visit. Bill has family in Roscommon in Ireland he told us.

Dr. Bihari called us in and expressed sincere gratitude for my efforts in Ireland with regard to LDN and MS. He was receiving many phone calls from Ireland with reference to my name. He was very excited and told me that he was hopeful trials in Africa would start in February 2003 for HIV and AIDS.

Dr. Bihari also showed me a copy of a fax he received informing him that the question of an LDN trial for MS was recently raised in the Scottish Parliament. I asked him to make me a copy of that fax so I could investigate more. I told him that my wish was for a clinical trial in Ireland for LDN and MS and I explained that there were many people running with it in Ireland, not because of me, but because LDN seems to work for MS. I explained that the MS societies in Ireland are generally run by people with MS or a loved one afflicted, so they have a personal interest and were helping to get the word out.

I asked Dr. Bihari outright how far would he be willing to go to help get a trial get off the ground. I told him that my plan would be to get him on the airwaves first, then with the help of the media mount pressure on the government to take initiative. He said that he would do all in his power to carry out a clinical trial with a reputable body. He told me that he wouldn't charge anything to set up a trial. All he would ask for is basic flight and board. The only thing the government would have to pay for is the actual trial which he would set up free of charge, he explained. He estimated the cost of a trial to be about two million Euro at the time.

I could see and clearly remember feeling that Dr. Bihari genuinely feels for all of the families that could be helped by LDN, and that he desperately wants LDN to hit the masses before his time is up. What also struck me at the time was his lack of desire for any personal gain. It just did not seem to matter to him. I was honestly humbled by his humility because he wanted nothing in return except the scientific recognition of LDN so that it would hit the masses. I could not imagine how anybody could not like the guy.

Dr. Bihari proceeded with the consultation and examined Neilus. He concluded that not only did Neilus not decline, he had actually improved modestly. He said that Neilus' facial expression was much better and as soon as he said that I realized that was what I couldn't put my finger on at the airport. It was true, Neilus had more facial expression. Also, Dr. Bihari believed that Neilus' gait was swifter and his arms were less rigid.

Then Dr. Bihari shared with us that he had nine Parkinsons patients at that time on LDN and all were stable. Some had more improvement than others, he stated. Overall he was delighted with Neilus' progress. Neilus and I were so happy. Once again we were filled with hope.

Before we left his office, Dr. Bihari convinced me to start taking LDN because of Mom's breast cancer. He explained that because she was struck post menopause, the chances of me being at risk were reduced but if I were his daughter he would prefer me on it. I told him that I was waiting for something to happen first, but he told me that he would not mess around. He said that it is a very strong gene and that he wouldn't take any chances.

It is amazing how different my questions became once I was asked to take LDN myself. I told Dr. Bihari that my concern was that my body would become dependant on LDN for endorphin production and if ever I went off it I would plummet. He assured me that would never happen. He said if I took LDN my endorphins would be raised to their correct level and if I came off it they would just go back to pre LDN.

"Prevention is always best!" he said.

If my endorphins were low he told me nothing would raise them. He said again that they cannot come back up on their own. That meant that whatever I am genetically predisposed to acquire would show if my endorphin levels were low.

I had experienced sufficient stress in previous years to think that my endorphins could have taken a hit so I decided to start LDN. I have to admit I would have been more comfortable with a blood test proving to me the state of my endorphins but I started LDN anyway. I would also have liked the promise of a blood test after a few months on LDN that would prove to me that my endorphin levels had actually improved, but as I said before such a test is apparently not that straight forward. I think that such a blood test would greatly help. At least it would be a form of measurable evidence seeing as proof in improvements with MS is so elusive.

Chapter 23

Our house had plenty of LDN so I popped one December 17th before my prescription arrived. I woke at 2:00 a.m., completely alert and ready to start my day. I could not get back to sleep until about 4:00 a.m.. This lasted for about a week.

Since then I have noticed that my hair and nails grow faster, I sweat more and I need less sleep. The rapid hair growth and sweating are not the most endearing of feminine traits and are ones I would never want exaggerated or publicized but they are manageable and only I would ever notice. I have also noticed that it is easier to track my fertility on LDN because it seems to heighten the signs. I suppose I should really point out that Natural Family Planning is not something in which I have ever excelled, but LDN did help me to recognize the signs more easily. Overall, I feel good but I have always been blessed with good health so I am not any example as to whether or not the drug is really effective. However, these are all good signs in my mind that LDN is doing something positive.

Kate, Rosemary and I started LDN around the same time that Christmas. We exchanged e-mail daily to report on our progress and I enjoyed getting to know them. Rosemary had no problems adjusting whatsoever. Kate, like me had difficulty sleeping initially. We were wired for about a week and swore that we looked like we had been hit by a bus. It was fun though, because we were in it together and I was confident that it would pass as I had been tracking LDN for some time. Kate and I adjusted, and started to sleep normally but her energy levels did not come back and I felt dreadful about that. I felt that I probably raised her hopes too high with my optimism.

I could not understand why she did not seem to be responding to LDN and I found it difficult to accept. Then, thank God, Kate announced that she was pregnant. She and her family were ecstatic. It was wonderful news. Dr. Bihari advises his patients to come off LDN for pregnancy, although he has some patients with AIDS who remained on it for the duration and had healthy babies. Until the drug is clinically proven he recommends to play it safe. Kate stopped taking LDN towards the end of January 2004 and gave birth to a beautiful baby boy, Matthew, on October 14th. She was Dr. Bihari's first Samters patient but she was not on the drug long enough to prove or disprove its effectiveness for Samters. Kate intends to resume LDN after she finishes breastfeeding Matthew. Thank God also, Kate had a remarkably healthy pregnancy. She is delighted with motherhood, a complete natural by all accounts, and her excitement is quite contagious. I so hope that when she resumes LDN, it will work for her.

The problem with Samters and all autoimmune diseases, as I have already stated, is that there is no effective treatment, except steroids to mask the issues and antibiotics to deal with recurrent infections, both of which have long term side effects, especially if over used. It would be wonderful for all Samters patients if Dr. Bihari is correct in thinking that LDN would be an effective treatment.

It is also worth mentioning that at present there are some very hopeful MS medications in the pipeline, in particular goat serum injections and stem cells. What is remarkable about LDN is the wide range of diseases it seems to help. It just threads them together. That is why a trial would shed some much needed light on how the immune system actually works. I also think that LDN would only compliment goat serum injections and stem cell therapy. It is very likely that it would make such promising treatments even better. The more I think about it, an LDN trial is simply imperative because it holds far too much promise to ignore.

After we celebrated Christmas and rang in 2004, Mom, Dad, Annie and Neilus flew back to Ireland and I decided to follow up with

Pat Kenny and investigate what was going on with the Scottish Parliament. There seemed to be so much happening and it was exciting.

Rosemary shared my interest. She used the internet to keep up to date with what people were saying about LDN. I loved conversing with her and e-mailed her regularly. It amazed me how easily I could open up to her on all levels. She said that she enjoyed our connection and looked forward to hearing from me, so a friendship developed that I will always enjoy.

I actually learned how to channel my enthusiasm for writing to Rosemary into this story, which will hopefully entice people to investigate LDN, either for themselves or a loved one. If more people investigate then more people will help everyone currently involved with the efforts for a clinical trial by putting pressure on the various Governments through the media most likely. If I manage to publish the story and pay off a mortgage payment, all the better.

Better yet, maybe the story will grant me some celebrity status that I can use along with my newfound wealth to actually privately fund a trial. That may seem difficult and sound a touch overly optimistic but it may be easier than attracting the attention of current celebrities. I never realized how difficult it actually is to get the attention of a celebrity. How many crazies can there possibly be out there bothering them all on a daily basis?

I started with Pat Kenny, a popular TV broadcaster in Ireland. The story in my mind seemed right up his alley. I thought that he would even thank me for bringing it to his attention. I sent him a follow-up letter late January 2004 but he didn't respond. I still can't believe that despite my persistence, he has managed to ignore me.

I have nothing at all against Pat Kenny or any celebrity whom I tried to entice because in my mind the sorry truth is that LDN lacks credibility. I cannot blame anyone with power to influence and personal credibility to maintain for treating the matter somewhat dubiously. It requires someone somewhere with position and power to take a leap of faith. But, as time passes the leap is getting smaller and smaller as the anecdotal testimonies multiply. I still believe that in time, Pat Kenny will run some sort of a story on LDN.

The initial letter that I wrote to him in September 2003, did serve much purpose though. If I had known at the time that the letter I was writing was going to be widely circulated I would have put more effort into it but it went as follows:

Subject: Multiple Sclerosis
To: todaypk@rte.ie
Date: Thu, September 25, 2003 12:18 pm
Dear Mr. Kenny,

My name is Mary Bradley. I live in New Jersey, USA and have a story I would really like the Irish public to hear but am not sure how to go about this. I would appreciate your opinion.

I am thirty-two, my husband is thirty-six. We have three little girls aged five, four and nearly three. My husband has had MS for about ten years. He was officially diagnosed in September 1998 during his first major relapse in London. We moved to New Jersey in January 1999 and in July 1999 he began Avonex therapy which is a standard form of treatment for MS patients. It is an injection taken once a week. At that point he was numb from the waist down but could walk unaided after he taught himself how to walk with the new loss of sensation. He never regained any of the sensation but we proceeded with our lives and were happy with the Avonex in that although he obviously slipped yearly, in that his stamina and ability to walk certain distances kept decreasing, we felt we were doing something and were beating the odds.

Then came January 2002. He just started to slip fast. He became very dependent on a cane whenever he left the house. Then came March 2002, he became dependent on his cane at home. He took steroids in May 2002. They pulled him back a bit for a short while but by August 2002, he could hardly get off the couch, kept falling over and watching him climb the stairs was frightening. I was going to get him a walker for the house and move our bedroom downstairs. He tried steroids but they didn't work. His neurologist really wanted him to continue on the Avonex or switch to Copaxone (a daily injection) as there was nothing else to offer. Things were grim.

Then I found a doctor in New York City. This doctor, Dr. Bihari, claimed that he had seventy patients with MS all in remission, some with huge improvements, taking one pill a night, with no side effects. His first patient is his daughter's best friend on this for seventeen years with no progression. Also this drug is cheap, $35 a month and FDA approved at much higher doses. It all sounded too good to be true. We took the information to the neurologist and he said that there is no way it could work but agreed that it also could do no harm. To humor us he prescribed it. My husband came off the Avonex and started LDN 4.5mg nightly September 12th 2002. Within six weeks he could walk normally again with his cane. He stopped falling over and we had our lives back. It is over a year now and he is still walking normally with a cane, not falling over, no relapsing and no need for steroids. It still seems too good to be true.

Dr. Bihari believes that everyone with MS has low endorphin levels. Endorphins regulate the immune system. He claims that LDN (Low Dose Naltrexone) if taken between 9:00 p.m. and 3:00 a.m., triples endorphin production. When this happens the immune system cannot attack itself anymore. MS is an autoimmune disorder whereby the immune system attacks the myelin sheath of nerve endings. This causes scarring of the brain and spinal cord. Dr. Bihari believes that the LDN will only reverse recent scarring, that which occurred within the last three months but he claims that MS will not progress. It is emotionally dangerous to fully believe this but so far he is right. I cannot help but believe. My husband refuses to believe it will hold his MS at bay forever but also says that if it all goes to pot in the morning he had a good year!

Because of Dr. Bihari's success with MS he started reaching out to other autoimmune disorders. My uncle from Donegal flew out here to meet Dr. Bihari September 2002. My uncle has Parkinsons. He became Dr. Bihari's fourth Parkinsons patient and one year later, he has not progressed. It is shipped to him every three months from Irmats pharmacy in New York City.

I have a friend in Galway whose husband has MS. He is Robert and was also on Avonex and getting worse. I told them my story. He went to his neurologist in Galway who told him to give LDN a try. It is not compounded in Ireland so Robert had to get it on his own. He found Dr. Lawrence in Swansea who has MS himself and is taking LDN from Dr. Bihari in New York. Robert is getting his LDN shipped from Dr. Lawrence. His details are ...

Dr. Bob Lawrence,
Dietry Research Ltd,
10 Heol Gerrig,
Treboeth,
Swansea SA5 9BP. Tel:01792 417514
E-mail:bob.lawrence@ntlworld.com.
http://www.msrc.co.uk/index.cfm?fuseaction=show&pageid=625

Robert is doing incredibly well and wants to bring this to the national papers and I hope he succeeds. He is on this about two months now and his fatigue is practically gone.

There are now over 2,000 people here with MS, all in remission, some with more improvements than others. There are many LDN message boards on the internet. The www.ldninfo.org has a link to one, and another is http://www.voy.com/156761/.

I have tried posting my story on the MS Ireland webpage, and many other MS Sites, but it is constantly blocked. I have contacted the MS Societies in Ireland by phone, namely, Aidan in Galway, Chris in Dublin, Elizabeth in Cork, John in Letterkenny to name but a few and they are all keenly interested and investigating. Some have MS or a loved one with MS.

It is important that LDN isn't broadcast as a cure or over inflated, as to play on the emotions of people with MS is not right. However it would be wonderful if all with MS had access to this information and made up their own mind as to how to treat their illness. To get the drug approved for MS will cost millions and it is a very cheap Drug already approved at much higher doses (50mg) so nobody is going to make money on this and most with MS don't have enough time to wait for this. If it is agreed that the drug cannot do any harm and does not cost an arm and a leg, surely it is worth a try. If it fails, it fails. The medications on the market for MS are very costly and have huge side effects and only promise to slow down progression 35% of the time. There really isn't an effective treatment for MS yet and MS is rampant in Ireland.

It really is food for thought. I would be delighted to hear your opinion and input as how to handle this story.

Yours Sincerely,
Mary Bradley

As well as sending the letter to my list of MS contacts in Ireland, I also e-mailed the letter to friends and family all over Ireland. It was probably the first insight many had in to our lives with MS and it touched some people deeply. Some people just ran with it. I remember Noel's dad called me to ask if he could give it to the doctors he knew in Donegal because he felt moved, after reading it. Friends in Ireland, whom I hadn't really talked to in years printed out copies and literally distributed them to strangers on the street. I laughed one day I logged on to the internet because a guy I never met from Letterkenny got my e-mail from the MS society in Letterkenny in Ireland, and sent me a copy of the letter and inquired if I knew anything about it. I really felt as if word was getting out. The LDN website editor also e-mailed me to ask me if he could use the letter on the official LDN website. I agreed and it is there now. The website address is http://www.lowdosenaltrexone.org/

I should have shared with Noel that his story was on the internet but I didn't and a funny thing happened. Noel was still doing great on LDN. As always he was high on life, but his latest kick, was a serious urge to give back to the community. He decided to participate in the organization of a Christian retreat called Cornerstone, which he attended the previous year. His role was a witness speaker whereby he had to give an account as to how God helped him in life. He felt it would be a good thing to share his epiphany with people. During the retreat he got to know many people, one of whom told him that he read his story on the internet because his sister had MS. Of course, I knew this man's wife and gave her all of the information and asked her to pass it on to her sister in law. Noel came home and knew that it could only have been me that posted his MS story on the internet. He asked me about it and I confessed. Thankfully, the glow of Cornerstone saved me.

I often think of the witness speech that Noel delivered. He let me read it and it hit me very hard that it would be a nicer world if everybody had a bit more "Noel" in them. The speech told about his childhood in Belfast, his lonely experiences at boarding school and his depression in London. Then, it gave a brief and humble description of his epiphany and continued to describe his MS diagnosis and progression. It sounded like a pretty depressing existence by all accounts to any normal person, but when I read the last line I really could not believe it. He actually felt that he had to tell the guys that his life wasn't perfect! He even qualified that statement by sharing with them that he "still fights with his wife over stupid stuff." That was pretty inspiring.

Chapter 24

It was early 2004 when I came across an article in *New Horizon's* Winter 2003 issue, by the Brewer Science Library in Wisconsin. It was written by Christina White and titled "LDN Results for Multiple Sclerosis Patients." She stated that she first wrote about some of the dramatic results that Dr. Bihari had reported with LDN use five years previously. Her first article on LDN was titled "Only One Pill A Day Keeps Some Cancers At Bay" and it was published in *New Horizon's* Spring 1999 issue. Since then, this was her fifth article following up on LDN and very detailed. It included a reference to the Goodshape website and said that it was one of the first websites to post LDN information. Christina wrote that Goodshape heard about LDN from one of their subscribers who posted on his site and she said that Goodshape called her to discuss results with it for various diseases. She commented on how the word was spreading like wildfire through the web based MS Community and she printed many LDN testimonies and clarified that all of the results were anecdotal. It was a well written account in my book and it was good to see LDN in print again.

Shortly after reading that article I decided to investigate what was going on in Scotland. I read the information Dr. Bihari copied for me in December. It stated that on Friday 12th December 2003, LDN was formally addressed in the Scottish Parliament. That sounded very promising. I knew that a trial in Scotland would do just as good as one in Ireland.

A woman named Irene Oldfather asked the Scottish Executive what information it had regarding LDN in the treatment of MS and of current prescribing practices for LDN in Ireland and North America. She asked them to compare the cost of current therapies with the cost of LDN. She also directly asked whether they would consider funding clinical trials to monitor the effectiveness of LDN in the treatment of MS. That was what held my focus.

I posted on the Yahoo LDN message board to find out who was responsible for this. A couple named Lorna and Terry, from Scotland, replied to me in private. Lorna is in her mid forties and she started LDN to treat her MS in April 2003. She was so impressed with the results that she and her husband were trying as best they could to get the drug into a clinical trial in Scotland.

The first thing Lorna noticed on LDN was that the numbness in her back improved. Then her stiffness and fatigue also began to fade. One morning she got up, worked on her computer, cooked and tidied up and she was absolutely delighted with herself because prior to taking LDN she could not do anything before late morning. Lorna and Terry told me that they would update me as soon as they got word from the Scottish Parliament and I promised them that I would keep them informed of events in Ireland.

On January 13th 2004 the Scottish Parliament replied to the questions. Basically they said that they had no information on LDN and MS. They said that they were not directly funding any research, including clinical trials on MS. That was mainly due to the fact that no research proposals on MS had been received in recent years they claimed. They stated that they would be pleased to consider research proposals for innovative MS studies of a sufficiently high standard. They also added that these proposals would be subject to the usual peer and committee review. At least the Scottish Parliament was now aware of LDN I thought.

Meanwhile in Galway, Robert and others were organizing an LDN conference in The Menlo Park Hotel for January 16th 2003 at 8:00 p.m.. The event was advertised in the Galway MS Newsletter and broadcast on local radio. I informed Lorna and Terry, and they flew over at the last minute to attend. The conference room spilled out into the hall and Robert spoke to the crowd about LDN. Many people I know attended and by all accounts he gave a remarkable account backed by his wife. Lorna also told her story and I was told that she was a major asset to the event. After that conference more people got my e-mail from the Galway MS Society and the word continued to spread.

At this stage, a pharmacist in Gort, in County Galway, named Brendan was supplying LDN and he was starting to become inundated with queries. Also, Robert managed to persuade his neurologist in Galway to prescribe his LDN and the Western Health Board agreed to pay for it under the Long Term Illness Act. Unfortunately, Brendan also has a loved one affected with MS. He read everything on the internet about LDN and thoroughly investigated. Brendan does not like to accept something blindly and that is why he is a good pharmacist.

After much research he started to prepare LDN for people wanting to try it. For some he was making it up in liquid form and for others he was importing the capsules from Martindale Pharmaceuticals in the U.K.. He could see positive results but he could not explain them. We started to converse regularly and the more we talked, the more driven we became for a proper clinical scientific trial. The reports that I got back from people starting LDN kept me focussed. It was worth every effort.

It is important to point out that not everybody wanted to try LDN. There was then and still is now, a personal risk people feel that they have to take in order to try it. There always will be that feeling for some people until the trial is carried out.

Chapter 25

There are many people whom I love to keep in touch with in Ireland and I make a point of getting together with them every time I am home. One of these people is Maura. She was my hockey coach when I was in school and because we traveled so much together, we got to know each other very well and became good friends. I was always aware that her sister had MS. Shortly after Noel started LDN, I gave Maura all of the information on LDN and she passed it on, but her sister opted for chemotherapy instead. It turns out that the chemotherapy is actually working very well. However, it is not stopping her MS progress. The last I heard, she is considering the LDN on completion of the chemotherapy.

I was sorry to hear recently that Maura herself has developed a neurological problem that has confused all of her doctors. She has had a very difficult few years and is now considering trying LDN herself to see if it will help her. She would simply love to try LDN immediately just to see if it would offer her any relief but she lacks the energy at present to put the effort into getting the prescription. That is still not an easy task in Ireland by any means. I know that there are many Mauras in Ireland.

Actually I am pretty sure that there are many Mauras world wide. People who have educated themselves on LDN and clearly see that it is safer than aspirin, will not break the bank and has so much anecdotal evidence that they are desperate to try it but just can't. Many doctors are not willing to write a prescription for LDN and if they do they don't want it known. That is a crazy situation but also a reality. Doctors feel that they are putting themselves at risk of being sued because there have been no formal trials.

Patients in the U.S. have had to sign waivers stating that they will not hold the doctor responsible for whatever happens to them on LDN in order to get it prescribed. Some people have actually pretended to have a drug or alcohol problem in order to get a naltrexone prescription. Then they crush the naltrexone and add water themselves in order to home brew a lumpy nightly shot. But many people give up because they don't have the energy to fight the system or the confidence to home brew.

Thankfully, there are a handful of doctors who went to the trouble of investigating the drug and deduced it a safe prescription to write and are not afraid. If more doctors would investigate, more fear would be removed, but until there is a trial there will be a reluctance on the part of many doctors to seriously consider the benefits of LDN. That makes for an incredibly frustrating situation for too many people.

I know another lady, from the Mom's Group at Nativity. Her dad was a cop in Florida for most of his life. He is now retired, but for years they suspected that he had Lymes Disease. Then, in his mid fifties he was diagnosed with MS and told that there was no treatment for him to take. This happened not so long ago. His neurologist told him that he was too old for any of the MS therapies. Also, it sounds as though he has progressive MS because it is progressing rapidly. This lady has shared many horrific stories about her dad's near death experiences as a result of his MS, like falling head first through glass doors for example. She is deeply concerned for him but she cannot get him a prescription for LDN because his doctor has never heard about it and that is good enough for her dad. Like many, he wants to do what his doctor thinks is best for him. This drives his daughter insane. That is a very tough situation but I can understand her dad. It is by no means unreasonable to want to listen to your lifelong doctor.

On the other hand there is Rachel's husband's Aunt Ava in Pennsylvania. We visited Rachel and her husband in October 2003, shortly after they moved to Ohio. I made a point of meeting Ava who was visiting her sister in Ohio at the time because Mike told me that

Ava has MS. Ava is about fifty, she is blind and the distance she can walk is limited but she is very mentally alert.

There are fighters and then there is Ava. She has not had an easy life but she certainly makes the most of it and I believe that she inspires everyone she meets. She took all of the information I had and thoroughly investigated it. She followed up on everything and e-mailed me with many queries and concerns. Ava took the information to her neurologist and literally insisted on a prescription. She has a good relationship with her neurologist and he has respect for her judgement. She was on Avonex at the time and she made the personal decision which is never easy, to come off it. That made her neurologist very nervous but it didn't bother Ava once she made up her mind. LDN is not compounded in Pennsylvania so I taught her how to home brew. She ran it all by her pharmacist and she is still making her own. Her neurologist still wants her to go back on Avonex or Copaxone but she refuses. Although his neurological exams didn't pick up on any improvements Ava feels better within herself. She says that she is less tired and can walk around her house all day. She feels that LDN is working for her. I recently heard that she had an MRI two years after starting LDN and it showed no new lessions. Ava is glad that she discovered LDN. I think that everyone with an autoimmune disease who has discovered LDN is glad that they did.

By February 2004 I had no doubt that Dr. Bihari had discovered something with the potential to help millions but I still didn't see the whole picture clearly. I was so focused on MS it was as if I had blinkers on. My main focus was Ireland because the few MS Societies I contacted in the States instantly blew me off. They just didn't want to hear about LDN so I basically gave up on spreading the word in the States. I desperately wanted them to take the matter seriously, but I was hit with a pre-written response every time. My dealings with the National Multiple Sclerosis Society (NMSS) in the States have been very discouraging to say the least and I have stopped donating money to them. Cold and corporate is the only way I can describe them. Instead of them actively investigating what can only be described as over whelming anecdotal evidence as to the effectiveness of LDN for MS, they stuck their head in the sand and said that they cannot comment or help in any shape or form until the drug is clinically proven. Surely it is the duty of the MS Societies to help the fast growing web based MS community set the LDN record straight? If not, it should be. Maybe their name needs to be adjusted also in order to clarify their primary interests.

Sometimes, the enormity of the battle for a trial would get me down. It can be so frustrating and depressing to think that the battle is such an uphill struggle because of the lack of financial profit LDN holds. That is so wrong. It highlights something so wrong with the way the world works that it makes my blood boil. I basically gave up on the States because I could not see a large scale LDN trial entice any business to investigate and my focus became Ireland mainly because they stood to make money on the outcome of a successful trial.

I shared my frustration with Rosemary who knew what I was trying to achieve and for some reason understood me very well. She always kept it light and I enjoyed her gentle wisdom. There were times I think that I really needed it. She never agreed or disagreed with my perceptions but she always listened.

Then one day Rosemary told me that she thought that I needed a wider audience. She had seen an Oprah Special Report that Christmas about Aids in Africa and she remembered that Dr. Bihari was looking at doing a trial in South Africa for LDN and AIDS. Rosemary deduced that Oprah would be interested to hear about an LDN trial in South Africa, and that if Oprah became convinced of LDN's potential, then she would most likely do all that she could to help it reach the masses. I decided to investigate.

Chapter 26

I don't watch TV very much so I was not too familiar with Oprah. I knew very little about her but the more I read, the more I liked her and the more I understood what Rosemary was saying. It was clear that if I could convince Oprah of the potential LDN held for AIDS in South Africa, she would without question do all in her power to get it to the people. That would have to involve a scientific clinical trial, and if a clinical trial proved effective for AIDS and HIV by boosting the immune system, then I figured that the MS community leaders would have to sit up and take notice.

Oprah recorded a remarkable documentary on AIDS in South Africa and it was aired Christmas 2003. I imagine that she made her point with millions, me included. It was a human approach where she met and befriended real people dying of AIDS, leaving behind real children. Her main focus was the on the children and I think that anybody who saw the reality of the lives some people in South Africa live must think twice before ever complaining again.

The show was called Christmas Kindness and it took Oprah a year to make it. She hired one hundred people to get the word out that the children were invited to a Christmas party, and she brought along many gifts. She even referred to it as the single greatest experience of her life.

Oprah gave each child a pair of shoes and a photo of themselves. Each girl received a black doll, and each boy, a football and she also gave away jeans. She made Christmas special for tens of thousands of children from the most wretched of villages far too familiar with death.

From an interview Oprah did with Diane Sawyer, I learned that every minute in South Africa, sixty-four people die of AIDS. They have left behind a whole generation of children without parents, food or any way out.

There may be as many as eleven million of these orphans, according to the United Nations. It's as if every child under the age of nineteen in New York were left to raise themselves. It is absolutely tragic.

South Africa's president, Thabo Mbeki, had long described poverty as the biggest threat and killer in South Africa and has expressed doubts, both about the link between HIV and AIDS and the extent to which the disease has spread in South Africa. But the South African government has now approved the provision of AIDS drugs to HIV positive people through the public health system. That was a significant step forward but they need more. They need LDN.

It was an unbelievable personal experience educating myself on the enormity of the AIDS epidemic. It hit me on a level I didn't know I could reach. The actual potential LDN possessed, according to Dr. Bihari slowly sunk in. It went so far beyond MS that MS actually seemed small in the grand scheme of things. My blinkers came off. I remembered everything Dr. Bihari told me about AIDS and HIV from when I first phoned him. I also remembered that he was very excited and eagerly anticipating a trial in South Africa for LDN and AIDS when I visited him in December. I had no doubt that Oprah would indeed be very interested.

At this point I really just wanted her to know about LDN regardless of whether the MS community leaders took notice or not. I also had no doubt that Dr. Bihari was right. I felt no reason to doubt him because what he was saying about MS and Parkinsons seemed to be holding true. If what he said proved to be true for AIDS and HIV, the implications were staggering. I began to get excited about the trial myself. His claims are difficult to believe but it comes down to one point in my mind, what if he is right? What if even half of what he says proves to be true? In my heart I do believe he is right but the question has to be, how right is he?

Dr. Bihari claims that 4.5mg LDN actually prevents HIV developing into full blown AIDS if the patients CD4 count is greater than 300. How unbelievable is that? Although as stated earlier, his early work consisted of helping those afflicted with drug and alcohol abuse, in the 80s his work extended to the HIV and AIDS community. He published a paper in 1986 that was presented in 1988 to the International AIDS Conference in Stockholm, Sweden. His paper described in detail a placebo controlled LDN HIV/AIDS clinical study. He is currently following twenty patients with HIV who over many years have refused antiviral drugs, but continue to remain healthy on LDN alone. Also, in 155 patients with AIDS treated for the past four years by using LDN in addition to antiretroviral therapy, Dr. Bihari found that over 90% continue to show no detectable level of virus. This is a substantially higher success rate than for any reported AIDS treatment group. In addition, these patients have not developed the side effects like lipodystrophy, which occur without LDN use.

I cannot deny that it sounds too good to be true but it gets even better. With local manufacture in South Africa, LDN would cost no more than $10 per patient per year. And finally, without wanting to sound like an LDN commercial but because LDN is a simple pill taken nightly, if clinically proven, it would hold great advantages over the combination antiviral regiments. Namely, it can be taken with discretion, which is a big plus given the cultural stigma that accompanies AIDS and HIV victims, and it has no side effects or need of medical supervision. These are life saving advantages for South Africa. It certainly sounds like a wonder drug, but by all accounts it is a wonder drug worth investigating because the promise it holds is literally phenomenal. I cannot help but constantly wonder exactly how right is Dr. Bihari?

Once I had the picture clear in my mind, I set out to write Oprah a letter. Before I did that I read her biography to try to figure out what she was all about. It is only as I write this story do I realize that I have a unique way of approaching situations. I figured that she must be bombarded with mail, so Rosemary suggested I call Dr. Bihari to ask him if he could give me anything to make my letter stand out.

Dr. Bihari had seen Oprah's Christmas Special and thought at the time that it would be wonderful if she knew about LDN. He told me that he had a great deal of respect for Oprah and all the work that she was doing in South Africa. He was very appreciative of my efforts and delighted that Rosemary prompted me. He remembered her from Kate's Samters consultation in December. He did warn me that he had tried in the past to contact various celebrities and he concluded that it was by no means an easy task.

I asked him if he would tell me about the upcoming trial. He told me that there was a strong possibility that a trial was going to happen in Mali in February 2004 for LDN and AIDS and HIV. He was so excited that I could hear it in his voice.

The interest was sparked by a twenty-four-year-old from Mali studying to get his MBA in Chicago who became familiar with Dr. Bihari's work. His father is a man of position in the Islamic National Bank in Saudi Arabia, and good friends with the President of Mali. Dr. Bihari was told by the young man's father that the President had agreed to let him fly over and meet the planning commission to set up a trial. He was anxiously awaiting a letter from the President of Mali to confirm this. Dr. Bihari planned to get his visa and head over there as soon as the letter arrived.

I asked him what he thought would be the best way for me to approach Oprah, I asked should I wait until he got back and wondered if he would keep a journal or take pictures that I could use. He said that all I needed to get her attention in his opinion would be a copy of the letter he was waiting to receive from the President. He figured that would be enough to get her attention. He said that he would contact me as soon as the letter arrived and fax me a copy. I was very excited when I hung up the phone and could not wait to share his positive response with Rosemary. She thought that it was wonderful that Dr. Bihari was on board and she agreed that the situation was exciting. I set to work on the letter.

The letter basically asked Oprah to take a leap of faith in Dr. Bihari. It was clear to me even then that in order for his theories to be tested, somebody with power to influence had to take an enormous leap of faith. The letter gave a history of Dr. Bihari and went on to detail the promise LDN held for AIDS and HIV based on the 1986 placebo trial and his current patients. It told of the Developing Nations Project Dr. Bihari initiated to reach out to the developing world and ended with my family MS, Parkinsons and breast cancer stories with reference to my perception of Dr. Bihari's humble and compassionate character. I sent a copy of the letter to Dr. Bihari to make sure that it was medically correct and asked him if the letter had arrived from the President of Mali. At that time the letter had not arrived. It is January 2005 now and Dr. Bihari has been in recent contact with the President of Mali and is finally in the process of setting up a trial. I intend to bring Oprah up to speed on the exciting news.

In February 2004, I decided to send my letter to Oprah on its own. I asked her to bridge the gap between Dr. Bihari and South Africa. I have to say, whatever about Pat Kenny ignoring me, I outdid myself in trying to capture Oprah's attention. I cannot help but feel if ever I write a book that she wants to feature in her book club, I just may have to make her sweat for a second or two.

Of course I firmly believe that she will run some LDN story someday because I know many people have written to her since with their own LDN stories. I imagine that she is still researching the whole thing because I have learned that everything in life takes a great deal longer than I would like.

Before I mailed the letter, I sent it to a list of family and friends, all of whom contributed something. It was Valentines so I waited a couple of days until after the mail rush, I scanned in a family picture at the end of the letter to make it more personal, I added my e-mail address, wrote a cover letter and used apple green paper. To be so sad as to know that apple green happens to be Oprah's favorite color is one thing, but to be so obvious about it is another. I now think that I probably scared the woman.

I nearly scared her a lot more, because I was going to send her fifty copies of the same letter because she had just turned fifty and I figured it was an even number. I also hoped to hit a cross section of her staff in the hope that one would find it worth passing on. I imagined a room full of people going through her sacks of mail and I wanted fifty of them to read it. Rosemary put a halt to that crazy idea by suggesting that I test the system first instead of presuming that it was at fault. She wanted me to give Oprah the benefit of the doubt initially, which sounded reasonable so I did. Another friend feared that fifty letters would prompt a visit from the FBI for stalking. At the time I joked that even bad publicity was better than no publicity.

I turned a simple letter into "Operation Oprah" and there was great relief when I finally sent it. I mailed it direct to Harpo. Of course I didn't just mail it, I sent it express, priority, delivery receipt written confirmation and certified. The young man at the post office looked at me that day and said "Gee Lady, you must want tickets for that show real bad." I laughed and said yes. I was very happy with the letter.

About a week or so later I received the written confirmation in my mailbox and noticed that the letter was received by a lady named Ana. I called Harpo in Chicago and asked to speak with her. She told me that she receives all of Oprah's mail and sorts it. It is then reviewed by the next level of people and whatever they find interesting goes to the research team, and if the content passes research, then it is brought direct to Oprah's attention.

Ana told me that fifty letters would have annoyed her intensely. I asked her what would be the best way to try to get Oprah's attention. She told me to watch a show and to note the names at the end and mail the names direct.

The names don't appear in New Jersey so I called my cousin Sheila in Chicago. She told me that her husband went on the Oprah show with his construction company, Liffey Construction, a while back when Oprah was doing a show on how to build panic rooms. It turned out that Sheila had a list of Oprah's entire senior staff, so I sent them all a copy of the letter and followed up with a phone call. I ended up dealing directly with a lady called Layla in Harpo. Layla assured me that they have received the entire story and it is in review. I am sure that Layla will call me any day now.

Chapter 27

"Operation Oprah" developed into "Operation LDN." The AIDS angle completely consumed me for the next while and I thoroughly researched the South African Government. I read a great deal about Thabo Mbeki and wrote a letter to him. The letter was basically the same as the one I sent to Oprah except it lacked any emotional pleas. It was more of a business letter propositioning his government to look into Dr. Bihari's work because it seemed to hold enormous potential for their country. I also sent the letter to a cross section of the South African government in the hope that one of them would take heed. As well as sending the letters in the mail I also e-mailed them. Once again as I write, it is obvious that the whole thing consumed me.

I was delighted and shocked to receive a prompt e-mail response from the South African government. It was from Charmaine Fredericks and dated March 23rd, 2004 and it read:

Dear Ms Bradley

We hereby wish to acknowledge with thanks receipt of the correspondence for the Deputy President regarding the work of Dr. Bernard Bihari.

This has been forwarded to the Deputy President's Special Adviser, Mr. Siyabonga Mcetywa who will liaise with you in due course.

For your information, Mr. Mcetywa's contact details are:
Tel.: +27 12 300 5310 Fax +27 12 323 3114

Yours sincerely
Administrative Secretary

That was exciting. I called the number in the letter and spoke with Mr. Mcetywa's secretary, Doreen, for about half an hour. She seemed very interested and assured me that she would pass on the information. I also received written confirmation in the mail dated May 13th from the Trade and Industry Ministry acknowledging receipt of the information with gratitude. That was also exciting. It is not everyday I get mail from a Government. I was delighted that at least they had the information. That is however the last I heard from South Africa.

I forwarded all correspondence to Oprah and her staff in the hope that she would take action but I am still waiting. It is not easy to interest a celebrity, any celebrity, and I know that.

I developed the "more the merrier" approach. I decided to tell as many celebrities as possible about LDN, focussing on those that openly care about the AIDS epidemic. My compulsion was contagious and my friend Coirle in Ireland, joined my efforts and starting pumping out letters herself. She also kept LDN information that she downloaded from the internet in her car so that when she was driving around Galway she always had a print out available for people she knew would have interest.

Also, here in New Jersey, the Mom's Group kept their eyes open and dispensed LDN information at every given opportunity. One day, a friend of mine called me on her cell phone from a pet store in New Jersey after she discovered that the owner had MS. It was a crazy thing for my friend to do and I really laughed afterwards, but she did put me in touch with the lady who was very grateful and most interested in the information. I was delighted. It was wonderful to have so much support from friends and family. That felt great.

I wrote to Bono, Mary Robinson, Bishop Tutu and Nelson Mandela in the hope that someone would eventually have their curiosity piqued and carry the torch. It seemed almost incomprehensible to think that no one would take the time to check it out but nobody replied.

On March 31st 2004 I wrote to the Bill and Melinda Gates Foundation. Rosemary noticed an article in the local paper that stated he had an online application form for research grants to help the AIDS Crisis. I found the application form and it seemed perfect for LDN. It was perfect because it was brief and straight to the point. I called Dr. Bihari to inform him and again he thought it worthwhile. I asked him how much I should request. His reply once again amazed me. He said that all that he would need to get a trial in South Africa underway was $250,000. I applied for the grant but was refused. I respected how prompt they were with their reply. On April 1st 2004 I received a letter of rejection from Bill and Melinda. Part of it read:

We agree that the work you describe will help to improve health in the developing world. However, it has been determined that the proposed activities are not among the current priorities for support by the Bill & Melinda Gates Foundation as our focus is on prevention rather than treatment at this time. In order to stay focused on our highest priorities, we must unfortunately decline funding for many worthwhile projects.

It is funny, but when you really look at it, the world isn't that big and I was quickly running out of options. On the MS front, I e-mailed Meredith Viera after a couple of friends prompted me to. They read her husband's story in the local paper. I also fired off the same letter to Montel Williams but once again nobody replied.

On the Parkinsons front I tried Michael J Fox but he didn't answer. I finally concluded that I needed to change tactics. Writing to celebrities although worth a shot, seemed futile.

Chapter 28

My daughter Annie's kindergarten spring break was approaching and I asked Noel if he wanted to take a trip back to Ireland but he couldn't because his work was very busy. He gave me the go ahead to make the trip with the children if I wanted to, so I booked our flights to Ireland for April 23rd 2004, for nine days.

On April 18th, my friend with MS from the Mom's Group organized a team to do an MS Walk in Ridgewood, to raise funds for the NMSS. I was reluctant to participate but I wanted to show my personal support for my friend so I went along. The weather was beautiful and we all gathered at Graydon Pool in Ridgewood, New Jersey.

I could not contain myself when I saw all of the different teams and all of the people directly affected by MS. I wrote out the LDN website along with my name, address, phone number and e-mail on fifty pieces of paper and ran to each team and distributed it to the members. I explained the theory to most. I was delighted to have the support of two good friends from the Mom's Group for the walk. I wasn't sure if I was brave enough to approach complete strangers but they kept the pep talks running, pinpointed the targets and made it happen. I am still in touch with five people from that day with MS all of whom have started LDN and are doing great.

There was so much happening regarding MS and LDN on the internet at that time. It was very exciting. Many people were putting in tremendous personal effort to get the word out and help others. There were so many people reaching out and sharing personal but wonderful stories and experiences. The MS community really had momentum.

A lady named Edwina from Cork, joined forces with Robert in Galway, Lorna and Terry in Scotland and another lady named Linda in England, and together they put together an internet petition for people to sign asking for a clinical trial of LDN and MS. To date the petition has nearly 6500 signatures. When enough are gathered it will be presented to the Irish Government and others. The petition can be signed at http://ldn.way.to/

Edwina is in her mid-twenties and has relapsing remitting MS. I remember her from summer 2003 because I e-mailed her about LDN along with everyone else who had their details on the MS Ireland website. She investigated LDN, and when she decided to try it, she had great difficulty getting her prescription. She ended up getting it from Dr. Lawrence in Wales but had to wait quite a while for an appointment. Thank God, like Robert, she went on LDN and in turn has helped and educated numerous others. Fatigue and bladder control were the main improvements experienced almost immediately by Edwina.

As with Rosemary's daughter Kate, Edwina also conceived shortly after she started LDN. She was on LDN for six weeks when she discovered she was pregnant, and like Kate, she decided to stop LDN because she wouldn't feel comfortable taking any medication during pregnancy for fear it would harm her baby. Edwina gave birth to a beautiful baby girl, Ava, on January 20th 2005 and hopes to get back on LDN as soon as she can after breastfeeding. Edwina has her own website that she updates regularly at http://edwina.sail.to/

Meanwhile, Lorna and Terry were still campaigning on their own in Scotland and on April 12 2004, The Herald newspaper in Glasgow, Scotland, carried a feature article "MS Victim Finds Hope in Heroin Users' Drug; Campaign Launched for Urgent Trials of Naltrexone".

It mentioned the increasing number of people who are petitioning for clinical trials specifically people with MS, in order that LDN could be licensed for their use, and detailed a success story. That was all thanks to Lorna's efforts. I was delighted that she managed to get her story in the paper because I know that is not an easy thing to do.

As a group, the LDN campaign team are relentless in their efforts and determination to get LDN to all those that could benefit. Their priority is a large scale clinical trial. They are campaigning daily worldwide and when somebody finally takes the initiative to carry out a scientific trial, it will be in large because of the daily efforts of that group and many other similar alliances that have formed across the world as a result of LDN experience. I know that I am very grateful for the many wonderful people I have met through LDN.

Chapter 29

Before I flew home that April, I decided that I wanted to contact the Irish Government, but I knew at this stage that telling my story was not good enough. I needed to be able to tell them exactly what I wanted them to do and I figured out that I wanted them to do a clinical trial. They have everything to gain with the successful outcome of a trial so it made sense. I called Dr. Bihari and asked him if he would draw up a trial proposal for the Irish Government for LDN and MS that I could take to Ireland and present to them. As always, Dr. Bihari was more than willing to help. He agreed and thought it a sensible plan. The proposal wasn't ready before I flew so he agreed to fax it to me when I settled.

On April 23rd 2004, I flew to Ireland with my girls. They love to travel and are so easy to manage. They had their own luggage and they even packed it themselves. They felt all grown up. The journey was fun. They are out of diapers, bottles and pacifiers, so compared to previous trips, it was relaxing. We arrived in Shannon and were greeted by Mom, Dad and Annie. As always, it was a fun visit.

The whole family gathered in Renmore at Mom and Dad's house. All of my brothers and their wives and children and my Aunt Kathleen were there. I met my two new nephews, Ethan and James, and my first niece Christina. By now, Phil had married his perfect woman Evana, and Pat had moved home from London and married his, Karen. Mom had a path worn out to the Poor Clares but succeeded in gathering all of her sons around her to settle. My distance keeps that path fresh.

It was wonderful to see them all. Mom and Annie cooked a fantastic meal and when we were sitting around after, Pat asked me what my plans were. I told them that I wanted to go on radio because

I wanted to tell everyone about LDN. At first everyone laughed because they thought that I was joking.

I assured them I wasn't and told them that I wanted them to help me. Between all of them and their friends somebody had to have some connection with radio I thought. Then, my Aunt Kathleen rattled off a number, "double seven, double zero, double seven", she said.

Everyone looked at her and she repeated the number and said that I should call it first thing Monday morning and ask to speak with Keith Finnegan. We all cracked up laughing and teased her for knowing the number off by heart. Too many comical references were made as to why she would know such a number until she confessed that she went on the show to point out the different petrol prices across the country. It bothered her, and rightly, that prices are not uniform.

Aunt Kathleen liked the way Keith handled the story and told me that he was very down to earth and a popular broadcaster. My brother Vince said that I should try Gerry Ryan, a popular national Irish radio presenter. He said that he found Gerry very helpful one Christmas when he needed a turkey recipe. I laughed at the thought of Vince cooking Gerry's turkey. Dad asked Mom and Annie if Vince hurt their feelings by asking Gerry for the recipe. He asked them a couple of times but I don't remember a response. After a comical discussion about radio, I decided that to want to go on radio to talk about LDN was perfectly normal. They all wished me luck with Keith who we agreed in the end was the most sensible target.

First thing Monday morning I called Galway Bay FM and asked to speak with Keith Finneagan. A lady named Fionnuala answered the phone and asked me for my story. She said that she was in charge of gathering potential stories and advised me to e-mail her immediately. She assured me that she would review it and pass it on to Keith if she thought that it would interest him. I logged on to Dad's computer and hammered out the story and appended Mom's cell phone number.

Then I hit the road with the children to head for Donegal. Mom and Annie followed me in a car behind. Before we hit Sligo, which is about two hours from Galway and half way to Donegal, Fionnuala called me on Mom's cell phone. She loved the story and said that they would run it without a problem. I couldn't believe it. She asked me if Brendan and Robert, whom I had mentioned in the story, would be willing to participate. She explained that they would make the story more plausible because Robert is actually on LDN and Brendan is the pharmacist preparing it in Galway. I assured her they would oblige and told her that in order to make the show really credible we needed Dr. Bihari. She asked me if I thought he would be game. I was positive that he would play so I asked her to phone him and give it a shot.

I intended to phone Robert, Brendan and Dr. Bihari to let them know what I was doing but I lost my signal on the road so they all received a call out of the blue from Galway Bay FM, but they figured it out fast. Everybody was game and the show was scheduled for Friday April 30th at 11:10 a.m.. I called Dr. Bihari after everything was set and he assured me that he was delighted to participate.

After a wonderful visit with Noel's parents in Fahan, we headed to Arranmore Island to visit Grandpa Neilus. He looked wonderful. He still had a healthy glow about him and he was still able to weld and work twelve hour days if he had to. His Parkinsons was in remission without question.

I love visiting Arranmore and catching up with people I grew up with. Angela is a good friend of mine and as we caught up I shared with her that I was pretty sure that I was pregnant. She thought it funny, as did I. She assumed that a potential pregnancy implied that Noel was keeping well which pleased her.

After a short visit on the Island, the children and I began our journey back to Galway on Thursday April 29th with Mom and Annie a step behind. We all stopped in Letterkenny and I picked up a pregnancy test when Mom and Annie ran off somewhere with the girls. That was such a crazy day.

As only I would probably do, I took the test in a local pub, just because it was beside the pharmacy and I was in a rush to get back to the car to get on the road for Galway. The test was positive. I was pregnant. I laughed and called Noel. He was elated. He was so excited that he could hardly contain himself. He wished me luck for the radio show in the morning and told me that he would listen to it on the internet.

At that point the radio show was the farthest thing from my mind. I headed to the car. I immediately told Mom and Annie that I was pregnant and they instantly started planning another trip to New Jersey for the birth. I think that they were afraid to ask me how I just found out, but I told them what I did anyway. I made Annie laugh out loud and forced my Mom to pretend that she didn't hear me. That happens a lot with us. They were both very happy with the unexpected news.

I can't help but think that maybe my brother Phil is correct in thinking that LDN boosts fertility considering Kate, Edwina and I all conceived quite quickly after starting LDN with very little effort.

Vince's wife, Helen, called me on the road to Galway to tell me that I have the longest pregnancies because I tell people so soon. She said that most people at least wait until the test dries before announcing. I laughed because it was true.

Chapter 30

Dr. Bihari faxed me his proposal for an LDN trial in Ireland for MS the next morning shortly before the radio show. It was very interesting. Part of it read:

The autoimmune disease in which LDN is used most at present is Multiple Sclerosis (MS). Dr. Bihari currently has 384 patients with MS in his medical care in a private practice setting in New York City. These patients have been on LDN for an average of 2.5 years with a range of one week to nineteen years. The overall results of treatment with this drug have been excellent. Only three of the 384 patients have shown any attacks. To be more specific, one of these three, who started LDN eighteen years ago, at the age of twenty-two in 1988, had one attack after five years on the drug, thirty days after stopping it. The patient resumed LDN when the attack appeared and has had none in the thirteen years since. The second of the three, a forty-one-year-old woman had an episode of optic neuritis which cleared in four weeks, after eighteen months on LDN. The last of the three was a patient who experienced an episode of numbness in the left leg after eight months on LDN, not previously present, which cleared after three weeks. The other 381 patients with MS have had no sign of disease activity since starting LDN.

It went on to state that there are at present several thousand people with MS on LDN, who have had their LDN prescribed by their physicians after reading about it on the LDN website. It then proposed a twelve month placebo controlled study of LDN at 3.0mg. It recommended a sample size of 300 patients, 2/3's on the drug and 1/3 on placebo and estimated the cost to be less than 1 million Euro.

I presume that estimate did not account for MRIs but it all sounded very reasonable and enticing.

Robert phoned me that morning to meet for coffee before the interview. I laughed when he congratulated me on my pregnancy because it reminded me of how fast word spreads in Galway. It was of course his sister-in-law, and my friend, Coirle, who updated him. That was the first time I actually met Robert and I found him very relaxed and warm. We headed to the studio and I wasn't nervous at all because I didn't have time to think about it all week. Actually, I was so distracted for the week that I really didn't prepare, so when I put on the headphones, the nerves really hit me and I had to clear my throat a couple of times to combat them until I warmed up.

Overall the show went very well. I think that everybody I know in Ireland tuned in and the response was overwhelming. People all over the world tuned in because I posted on some LDN websites that Dr. Bihari was going to speak on the radio and they could hear it live from the Galway Bay FM website. Edwina followed up my post with instructions for all to follow if they wanted to hear the show.

Robert gave a very relaxed and compelling personal account of his LDN experience and Brendan stated very clearly that he was sure that Dr. Bihari was on to something as he was seeing LDN work for people in Ireland. Dr. Bihari explained LDN in terms that everyone could understand and relate to. His manner was confident, but also laid back. He was in no way pushy, just matter of fact and genuine. I know that he struck a cord with many. He shared that he and his wife were taking LDN as a cancer preventative for twelve years and he listed all of the cancers that he believed LDN would effectively treat or prevent. Dr. Bihari listed a number of illnesses for which he also believed LDN held potential, including alzheimers, rheumatoid arthritis, Parkinsons, sarcoidosis and lupus. He assured people that after many years on the drug his blood work was normal proving that LDN is a safe drug.

By all accounts the Keith Finnegan Show was a big success for LDN. It is funny, family members whom I had tried to explain LDN to for a long time finally got it and wanted to try it. Actually, most of my school friends also finally understood and the word started to spread again like wildfire. I joked that the next time I want my family and friends to hear what I have to say I will have to call Keith. Soon after the show, I was quickly inundated with e-mail again and only too delighted to respond.

The day of the radio show, Lorna called Robert to say that she heard the show on the internet and told him that she thought that we did a fine job. That night I met up with a couple of school friends who could not believe that I didn't broadcast my pregnancy. We went out for dinner and laughed about the radio. I told them that the funniest part of the whole thing was Mom. She was reversing into the drive in Renmore when she heard me on the car radio and she rammed the car into the wall and took off the back bumper. I laughed when I saw it and assured Dad that I was positive that it looked worse than it was, a common phrase in the Boyle household guaranteed to aggravate.

A good friend of mine in Galway is a nurse and she lined up a couple of phone calls to people she wanted to know about LDN. Another friend said that she wanted to start on LDN immediately for peace of mind. It was great.

I stated on the show that I was going to send the trial proposal to the Irish Government so I was keen to follow up on that. I didn't have time when I was in Ireland because by the time the government offices opened that Monday I was due to fly back to New Jersey, and thank God I had no idea what lay ahead

Chapter 31

We flew into JFK Airport on Monday, May 3rd. Noel met us at the airport in his wheelchair and I was so glad to see him. We are not very good apart. He was over the moon to see us, and the children climbed all over him talking in unison about their adventures in Ireland. Sara and Aisling resumed their normal positions, they sat on a knee each as he wheeled to the car. Annie holds the handles of the chair and she really thinks that she pushes them all. They are a happy sight and that is how they travel everywhere they go.

When the car was packed, Noel kissed me and we hung outside the car in the rain to catch up briefly. I told him that I felt great, that the children were so good for the flight and that we were going to have one memorable Christmas because the due date for the new baby was December 27th. He laughed and said that it would be our best Christmas ever.

Noel told me that I sounded great on the radio. Then he said that he managed to re-seed our back yard on his own, when we were away. He clarified that he nearly broke his neck many times in the process, assured me that the neighbors must think him crazy and admitted that he really is far too stubborn for his own good, but he swore that I was going to love it and think him brilliant. We joined the bedlam in the car and he drove us home.

After he put the children to bed, we made dinner and hung out for a bit to catch up. I was tired so I decided to take an early night. Things could not have been better.

I woke at 2:00 a.m. with severe cramping and nausea and assumed that I was experiencing morning sickness, because in Ireland it was 7:00 a.m.. I thought little of it initially. I remembered Mom telling my sister-in-laws whenever they were brave enough to mention morning sickness, that they were very lucky, because morning sickness is the happiest sickness there is. It is now commonly referred to as the "happy sickness" in the Boyle household.

By morning however, I feared that there was more to it, so Noel took the day off work and I went to the doctor. The doctor told me to come back for a scan at 3:00 p.m.. A friend from the Mom's Group, Stephanie, took our children, and Noel accompanied me for the afternoon appointment. Stephanie is a very close friend from the Mom's Group who will always drop everything to help me out. She is a very useful friend and renowned for her cell phone habit. Whatever the catastrophe of the day is, she flips out her phone like a flick knife and organizes the troops.

By the time I got to the doctor's office I was very weak and probably dehydrated so I passed out. They did the scan when I came round and confirmed that the pregnancy was ectopic and added that I needed immediate surgery because one of my tubes had burst and I was bleeding internally. I hated Noel being there for that. I so wished that he missed it, but there is no way that he would have. I will never forget the look on his face. I have never before seen a tear in his eye but I swear that I saw one that day. He got the fright of his life. For a second he really thought that I was going to die. He went from the happy expectant father to widower of three young ones in a split second and I felt dreadful for him. Then he snapped out of it and took control and brought me to the hospital. I think that he was fine when there was something for him to do, but once the doctors took over and hooked me up to everything I saw that look of fear return to his face. Thank God, another friend of ours, Kristen, works in the hospital. She came over to me and I told her that I was fine because I genuinely thought that I was, and asked her to make sure Noel was okay. She was wonderful. I will always remember her for being there.

When my blood pressure started to drop I asked the doctor to explain the situation to me. It was very sore. He told me that it was serious, and that they were trying to rush me into surgery as quickly as possible. He said that he didn't really know what to expect when they opened me up and he then took the liberty of explaining to me that ectopic pregnancy is the leading cause of death from pregnancy in the U.S.. I actually laughed when he said that and I told him quietly that my brother was a doctor in Ireland, and had a book with a chapter in it about good bedside manners that may be worth a look in his spare time. The nurse heard me and she laughed. I told Noel that there was a bright side, he could always write another witness speech for Cornerstone because this material was perfect. I was quite the comedienne.

When they were wheeling me in for surgery I really didn't know if I would wake up again. I realized that I had no control and I accepted that. I was positive that if my number was up then it was simply up and there was nothing I could do about it. I was surprisingly calm. I firmly believed that God would look after Noel and my children if I couldn't.

I was however greatly relieved when I woke up and informed that all went well. I only lost the tube that burst and I could go home the following day.

I was familiar enough with MS to know that she would not let recent events fade easily. I knew she would rear her ugly head as a result of the stress Noel experienced and I knew that LDN was about to be put to the ultimate test. I was on guard for the monster to attack and she did.

I was glad to get home to be with Noel and the children. I was also anxious to check my e-mail as I knew I had a lot of correspondence to catch up on from Ireland with regard to LDN. I was also eager to write to Rosemary. I was in constant e-mail contact with her, even from Ireland. She even listened to the Galway Bay FM Show on the Internet. I appreciated her support and I wanted to let her that know everything was okay.

My correspondence with Rosemary always helped me figure things out and put things in perspective. I never knew e-mail could be such fun. Annie was still in her class so had filled her in somewhat, but I wanted to fill in the blanks. I told her that I was going to send the proposal to the Irish Government as soon as I could and she suggested that I should learn how to crochet or needlepoint. As always, Rosemary remained balanced, neutral and light with a little affection. I knew that she was relieved I was okay. It is only now as I review our correspondence do I see how focused on LDN I really was for quite a period. I also realize that Rosemary helped me more than she will ever know.

I predicted an MS attack in an e-mail to Rosemary before it happened. This was not by any means fortune telling, just familiarity with the beast.

Chapter 32

Shortly after my miscarriage, I started to research the Irish Government. I found a website with a list of every TD and their e-mail address. On May 14th 2004, I sent Dr. Bihari's trial proposal for LDN and MS direct to the Taoiseach Bertie Ahern. I also sent a copy to the Minister for Finance, Charlie McCreevy and the Minister for Health at the time, Micheal Martin. Michael D. Higgins also received a copy because he used to lecture me in UCG. I also sent the proposal to various regional health boards who told me that it needed to be reviewed by Mr. Martin, the then Minister for Health. On May 19th I received the following e-mail from the Irish Government

Dear Ms Bradley

I wish to acknowledge receipt of your e-mail dated 14 May 2004 which will be brought to the Taoiseach's attention as soon as possible.
Yours sincerely,
Michael
Taoiseach's Private Office

I didn't get excited because I knew that an acknowledgment meant very little after dealing with the South African Government. It is just a courtesy.

On May 18th, Edwina and Robert managed to get LDN into the Irish Times. It read:

The Irish Times (Tuesday May 18th 2004)
Calls For Radical Treatment of MS

MS Sufferers in Ireland have begun a campaign for a clinical trial to be carried out on a radical treatment pioneered by a New York medic using a low dosage of naltrexone (LDN), a generic drug first licensed in the 1980s to treat heroin users.

About 6,000 people in Ireland have MS, a disabling neurological disease that interrupts "message traffic" between the brain and the body. Sufferers may lose muscle control, sight and experience fatigue.

LDN has apparently yielded positive results for neurologist Dr. Bernard Bihari of Beth Israel Hospital, New York, in halting the progression of MS and reversing its effects to a limited but, in some cases, significant degree for people with the more acute, progressive form.

LDN has also been used to treat different types of cancer and other auto-immune diseases such as HIV.

Once their petition is complete, the group, headed by Robert Joyce and Edwina Dennehy, intends making a submission to the Minister for Health, Mr. Martin, calling on a clinical trial carried out in Ireland, despite the negative implications for the leading pharmaceutical companies that produce the costly current MS interferon - 'CRAB' treatments, i.e. Copaxone, Rebiff, Avonex and Beta-Interferons.

Such MS Treatments are expensive and earn the drug companies massive profits. Witness the surge in Biogen Idec and Elan's share price back in February on the day when a new type of MS CRAB treatment—Antegren was announced.

Biogen Idec shares jumped $8.91, or 20 per cent, to %53.23, as of 4 p.m., New York time, in Nasdaq Stock Market composite trading, bringing the gain since the year began to 45 per cent. Elan gained 1.85 euro, or 27 per cent, to 8.77 euro in Dublin.

Joyce estimates these treatments are currently costing the Irish Government upwards of 24 million euros a year. Joyce believes that if LDN was licensed in Ireland, instead of an annual minimum medication cost of 12,000 euro per patient using one of the beta or *interferon treatments, the cost would fall to a fraction of this, with a month's supply costing less than fifty euros.*

Theoretically, however, the treatment flies in the face of conventional thinking on the underlying dynamic of MS—which effectively sees the erosion of the nerve channel's protective sheet - myelin - over time.

Instead of the erosion of the myelin sheet being caused by an over-active immune system, according to Dr. Bihari and advocates of LDN, the opposite is the case.

By administering low doses of the drug, which is an "opiate antagonist," an immune system deficiency triggered by a lack of secreted endorphins in the brain is reversed. This would open up the possible causes of the predominantly Western disease to such factors as lifestyle, stress and bad diet in addition to other possible causes - viral infection and genetic inheritance.

According to Dr. Bihari: "Up to the present time, the question of 'What controls the immune system?' has not been present in the curricula of medical colleges and the issue has not formed a part of the perceived wisdom of practicing physicians."

Nonetheless, he says a body of research over the past two decades has pointed repeatedly to the body's own endorphin secretion (our internal opioids) as playing the central role in the beneficial orchestration of the immune system, and the recognition of this is growing, he insists.

Support for this view was published in November 2003 issue of the prestigious New England Journal of Medicine.

The MS Resource Center in Britain is frank in its advise to patients: "LDN is a treatment method that has been in use in the U.S. since 1985 but is relatively new in this country. Despite its claimed successful use in America, until fully proven here, it must be considered as experimental and that no beneficial response can be guaranteed. In addition, despite the fact that the drug is very low dose, the absence of significant introductory or prolonged side-effects cannot be excluded."

It adds: "The treatment can only be provided if these conditions are accepted. Naltrexone is a drug, referred to as an opiate antagonist. Its normal use is to treat opiate drug addicts addicted to [drugs] such as heroin or morphine."

Its supporters in the medical profession say the brief blockade of opioid receptors between 2:00 a.m. and 4:00 a.m. that is caused by taking LDN at bedtime each night is believed to produce a prolonged "up-regulation" of vital elements of the immune system by causing an increase in endorphin and enkephalin production.

Normal volunteers who have taken LDN in this fashion have been found to have much higher levels of beta-endorphins circulating in their blood during the following days.

According to Joyce, he has seen a dramatic reduction in one of his main symptoms, fatigue, since taking the drug last August.

"I've found I have much more energy and was able to drive five hours from Oughterard to Valentia, whereas prior to beginning LDN I was exhausted on much shorter business trips in the passenger seat."

He said he first heard of the drug from a friend of his sister-in-law, whose husband also has MS and was seeing the prospect of using a wheelchair loom closer after prolonged attack.

"After a few weeks on the treatment he saw a marked halt to his progression and is still walking," he says.

However, the view from within the neurological establishment is less positive in the absence of clinical trials with hard scientific evidence gleaned from the much vaunted 'double blind trial' testing method.

One of the Republic's leading neurologists, Dr. Brian Sweeney of Cork University Hospital, refuses to entertain such anecdotal claims as a basis for prescribing the drug.

Dr. Sweeney says: "Without the scientific data backed up by a double-blind trial, where half the trial group are using a placebo and the other half are using the treatment, it's impossible to accurately say what the actual benefits of the drug administered in this way would be."

It is a view shared among his neurological colleagues in Ireland and MS Ireland, whose chief executive Michael Dineen says it will not be recommending the treatment based on anecdotal evidence alone. The organization's spokeswoman, Maura McKeon, adds: "Until trials are carried out on it, we cannot advise people to try this particular product. Up to now, we have received only anecdotal evidence of its effects."

While LDN is not licensed by the Irish Medicines Board (IMB), some GPs are prescribing it on an "experimental basis" when met with patient demands that they as doctors honour their Hippocratic Oath. But for the most part, the few Irish patients who are taking LDN, such as Edwina Dennehy, had to go through Welsh physician Br Bob Lawrence.

"I'm in my mid twenties and was diagnosed two years ago, having complained for several years of various symptoms such as fatigue, numbness and stiffness in my legs, etc. However, I found no benefits from the interferon treatments which, like many people, seemed to just make me feel worse," says Dennehy.

Disillusioned by the CRAB set of treatments and the growing feeling of her illness progressing, she has been very keen to get on LDN, having researched the treatment through the Web and heard of its benefits from Members of her MS mailing group. Her neurologist, she says, declined to prescribe it on legal grounds.

The problem, according to Joyce, lies in the fact there is no money for the big pharmaceutical players bringing on stream a treatment that already exists. "Naltrexone is now a generic drug and is past patenting, so it's not worth a pharmaceutical company's while spending several millions on trials and marketing of the drug, because it's already open season and any low-cost drug company from say India could come along and under-cut their market share in the global treatment of MS".

If LDN is to come into greater usage by MS patients, he believes it will most likely be from an Indian drugs company, which are beginning to develop their pharmaceutical sector quickly by manufacturing generic drugs much cheaper than their Western competitors.

In the meantime, the campaign to raise awareness of the benefits of LDN continues.

Dennehy set up an online petition for a trial to be carried out in Ireland.

She started her treatment over three weeks ago and says apart from initial disturbance to her sleeping pattern, she has found she has more energy and problems with her bladder have settled.

I sent that article as a follow-up to the same cross section of the Irish Government. I received an e-mail from everyone except Mr. Martin. They all said that it was Mr. Martin's job to review it and assured me that they forwarded him the information. My favorite reply came on June 11th. It read:

Dear Ms. Bradley,

The Taoiseach Mr. Bertie Ahern T.D. has asked me to refer to your e-mail of 9 June 2004 regarding your proposals concerning Multiple Sclerosis. The Taoiseach has forwarded your correspondence to his colleague Mr. Micheál Martin T.D., Minister for Health and Children for his attention. He has asked the Minister to have the points you raised addressed and to respond directly to you.

The Taoiseach has asked me to extend his best wishes to you.
Yours sincerely,
Nick Reddy
Assistant Private Secretary to the Taoiseach

It was a nice birthday present to have Bertie wish me well.

It is January 2005 now. Mr. Martin never responded. Mary Harney is the Irish Minster for Health now so I hope I will have more luck with her.

The ideal ending for this story of course would be that the Irish Government decided to start a large scale LDN trial for MS and LDN in Ireland, but a true story rarely ends ideally. The struggle continues and the snowball gets bigger every day. A large scale trial will happen though. It will happen somewhere. I do not doubt that.

I have questioned whether or not I should wait for a large scale trial to start before I publish my story, but I decided that many people don't have the luxury of time and my story may help somebody, somewhere, stop their disease in the nick of time. I don't want anyone to leave it as long as we did. What if Noel found LDN five years ago? Such thinking is too negative to dwell on, but there are many people at the stage Noel was at five years ago who can change their future. I really believe that, and I hope they do.

Chapter 33

Noel and I both felt a deep sense of loss after the miscarriage but an equally strong sense of gratitude for all that we had. We felt very fortunate to have three beautiful, healthy girls and each other, so we privately named the one we lost and moved on. At first things seemed fine and I wondered if I was just being paranoid or if the LDN was working better than even Dr. Bihari thought it would. Then came Noel's first relapse since starting LDN in September 2002.

I was mentally prepared for Noel to slip after the stress he experienced so I was not overly concerned about it. I was following people on the internet, in particular Goodshape's wife Polly. I knew that Polly slipped on occasion under stress or infection but she always managed to bounce back given time. I was very sorry to hear that on May 7, 2004 Polly died from heart failure at age sixty-five. Heart conditions seemed to run in her family, but she lived ten years longer than the average member of her immediate family. Her MS had been stable for four years on LDN and they were planning one more cruise that will never happen. Mr. Goodshape and Polly were married for 42 years and many felt his grief. He changed his website to focus more on LDN as he firmly believes that it is a miracle drug.

Reading about a relapse and watching one are two completely different things, and I can only imagine what it must have felt like for Noel to physically endure another blow. We were so spoilt for so long, even though his mobility remained greatly affected, LDN gave us much to be thankful for.

For the first time ever Noel actually got angry with his MS, and rightly or wrongly I got caught in the crossfire. Nobody was more convinced than me that we were going to live happily ever after and although he did all in his power to remain mentally prepared for a relapse, my constant optimism wore him down and he let his guard down. Noel was not mentally prepared to relapse. He got angry.

Then he got angry for getting angry. He hated not handling his decline with grace. He really had to readjust his focus until he found a way of dealing once again with an MS relapse. I cannot explain how awful I felt. I was responsible for his mental state in many ways.

My concerns went way beyond Noel very fast. I realized almost immediately that I had raised the hopes of many, many people who were more than likely in the course of their life going to experience sufficient stress or illness that would most likely cause them to slip. To slip when you are convinced you won't makes that slip much, much worse. It was a dreadful feeling and it hit home very hard that a level of responsibility is essential when dishing out medical advice without training on various websites when so little is really known about LDN. I always tried to qualify my advice with a note about my lack of medical training but I now realized that was not good enough. I realized that I don't know the whole LDN story or have all the answers. Without a clinical trial nobody does.

There are so many desperate people in desperate situations who really need LDN, but to reach the masses the right way it needs the backing of the medical community. I figured the only way to do all of the people justice and to maximize my time and efforts, was to fully dedicate my spare time to efforts for a clinical trial. That way everyone could embark on their personal LDN journey with their eyes wide open and the backing of the medical community to help them out in times of stress or infection. I want all the cards on the table for everyone to see, without illusion or false hope. That can only happen via a clinical trial of LDN.

I also felt at the time that there were many knowledgeable people posting on all of the LDN websites and guiding people, just as I was guided. It was around that time in July 2004, that I decided to write everything down and I have to confess the experience has been cathartic and therapeutic.

Although LDN is useful for a variety of autoimmune diseases the starting point in the trials should be MS in the developed world, because that is where the drug is used most at present, and AIDS/HIV in the developing world because of the promise it holds. From there it can be tested on the long list of other illnesses it seems to be useful for. Dr. Bihari is right, I do not doubt that he has found something worthy of a Nobel Prize, but once again just how right is he?

To describe Noel's relapse, it is obvious that compared to the whopper of 1998 this one was very mild. Dr. Bihari called it a pseudo relapse because Noel did not experience any new symptoms. He experienced a reoccurrence of old symptoms with an exaggerated vengeance. His upper body is still very strong and thank God the relapse only affected his legs. He never hit his worst point pre LDN. He always remained better than he was before he started LDN.

Dr. Bihari prescribed steroids for Noel and they worked a little for a short while. Noel remained on 4.5mg LDN while he took the steroids because Dr. Bihari thinks that although on paper they work against each other, in his practice he has found that it is not that straight forward. They seem to compliment each other in times of relapse. Noel also took the DL Phenylalanine supplement and felt that it also helped him a little initially, but not enough to keep taking it daily. I once again contemplated a walker for the house but Noel asked me to wait for a while.

It is January 2005 now and we rode the wave. His relapse ended about two months ago and looking at the overall picture he has lost some of what he initially gained from LDN although he may get it back yet. That is a shame because Noel really could not afford to lose anything. He purchased a home gym and has started to work out nightly in an effort to strengthen his legs. That is important for Noel because when he walks now, he doesn't use the muscles typically used for walking. His gait is different, so he has to exercise to maintain muscles that he no longer uses.

I took a really good look at Noel last night so that I could finish this chapter and I think that he looks very good. He doesn't fall over anymore, and he gets off the couch with little difficulty. I am no longer contemplating a walker for the house. He is without question better than he was pre LDN. That is the bottom line, despite the stresses life throws, after more than two years, Noel is still much better than he was pre LDN and he remains high on life. He never complains and is always fun to be with.

Even with LDN, MS still sucks but it is quite remarkable that Noel does not have any new symptoms since September 2002 despite massive stress at times. That gives me tremendous hope. LDN is the best treatment for MS currently available in my opinion because it does seem to stop progression. I know nothing for certain, but I hope and pray that Noel's MS never spreads any further. We can live very happily with our current hand.

On the Parkinsons front, my Uncle Neilus continues to work twelve hour days in the shipyards. His Parkinsons has also remained in remission since starting LDN in September 2002. His existing symptoms get worse with stress but he has not experienced anything brand new.

Also, it is interesting to note that after a review of his total clinical data through March 2004, Dr. Bihari reports that the use of LDN in some 450 patients with cancer — almost all of whom had failed to respond to standard treatments — suggests that more than 60% of patients with cancer may significantly benefit from LDN treatment. Sadly, my mom did not fall into that category. My family discovered in January 2005 that her breast cancer has spread to her bones. At present she is deciding her treatment options. Dr. Bihari is quite keen for her to try Metenkephalin. He is just starting to see that many of the cancers that do not respond to LDN alone, seem to be responding to LDN with Metenkephalin. I am still learning the theory behind his thinking but it is based on the LDN theory. Metenkephalin boosts the LDN effect according to Dr. Bihari. He is only recommending it for certain cancers at present. It is early days and my mom will decide her treatment, but she will be presented with every option out there so that she can make an informed decision.

When summer 2004 ended, my eldest daughter Annie started first grade. Aisling started Kindergarten and I am delighted that she is in Rosemary's class. Sara will not start Kindergarten until 2006.

Noel and I remain happily settled in New Jersey and have no intention of moving in the near future because it has become our home. We are delighted to be part of such a caring community. Thank God we have a wonderful quality of life.

Today, there is a fast growing worldwide grassroots movement working towards the scientific recognition of LDN. As more people experience the effects of the drug, the stronger this movement becomes. It is difficult to search the internet now for MS information without finding something on LDN. There are many LDN websites in many different languages.

There is an interesting informal LDN Survey on the internet that was filled in by 267 MS patients and the results concluded that LDN works better for MS than the approved medications. A lady named Samantha invested a great deal of personal time and effort to gather this information. This is a positive pointer that the LDN movement is heading the right way and I am certain that her efforts will greatly help towards a scientific trial. She created a website also at http:// www.ldners.org/ Everybody cannot be wrong. There is something in it and it holds tremendous hope.

There is a lot of wonderful news from around the world to report, but what the MS community needs is a large scale double blind placebo clinical trial for full scientific recognition that nobody can ignore. However these starting points are certainly worth celebrating.

In Ireland, Brendan, from Quinn's Pharmacy in Gort, has thirty people for whom he prepares LDN, Twenty-nine of whom have felt actual improvement. Many others in Ireland still import their LDN from the States or England, but that may change as Brendan has managed to get the Western Health Board to cover both the capsules and the liquid form. He is an avid campaigner and has happily helped many people acquire LDN. Brendan has also met with product development managers from Ranbaxy Pharmaceuticals and Pinewood labs to discuss manufacture and clinical trials, but as of yet there is nothing definite happening there.

I was most encouraged to see recently that Lorna and two friends of hers, Linda and Alex, got together in the U.K. and developed and registered an LDN charity. The internet address for this charity is http://www.ldnresearchtrust.org/ and the objective is to raise funds for an LDN trial and MS. They intend to start with MS and then branch out from there into trials for other diseases that Dr. Bihari thinks would benefit from LDN. I applaud their dedication and commitment and hope to come up with some way to help them. To date they have succeeded in convincing the U.K. MS society to help them get trials underway. They are also working very closely with Dr. Lawrence in Wales and a top neurologist in the U.K., and it looks like between them all, they have agreed to start two small trials. The first trial will prove that LDN is not toxic and the second will try to prove that it improves some small function such as bladder control in MS patients. After the successful outcome of the two small trials a large scale trial will hopefully be carried out. It looks most promising and I know that they are working around the clock to fund this endeavor via their website.

The local BBC TV news crew interviewed Linda in the U.K. on November 16th 2004. The registered charity faces the challenge of raising 35000 sterling pounds. That is what Dr. Lawrence and the neurologist estimate the cost would be for a one year toxicity trial involving twenty people. Should the charity succeed in raising the funds, Dr. Lawrence intends to start the trial in spring 2005.

A doctor from Ireland, Dr. Pat Crowley, flew to New York in January 2005 to meet and interview Dr. Bihari for Irish television. That interview will be broadcast on Irish TV and will also greatly help the LDN campaign.

I am equally excited about a group in Germany. A small LDN study started on October 15th 2004 in Hospital Dr. Evers, D-59846 Sundern-Langscheid, Germany and will continue until sixty participants are included. The goal of the study is to investigate what MS associated symptoms are positively influenced by LDN. When the results are compiled they can be viewed at http://www.klinik-dr-evers.de/

Also, an LDN trial for Crohn's disease is starting in the States. Jill P. Smith, MD, Professor of Medicine at Penn State's Hershey Medical Center, is enrolling patients in a four-month pilot study. This will test the effectiveness of LDN in offering relief to patients suffering from symptoms of Crohn's Disease and, if successful, should lead to a full-fledged clinical trial. The details of this study are maintained at the website http://www.hmc.psu.edu/colorectal/research/naltrexone.htm/

Finally, there is also talk on the internet about a University in Texas having interest in doing a small scale LDN trial for MS.

There are researchers in England, Australia, Germany and Italy investigating LDN and MS with great interest. All of this is happening because lots of people are putting much personal effort into spreading the word voluntarily, out of moral duty, because they have seen it work and empathize with desperate situations.

I am most eager to see the results of each study.

The only press coverage LDN received in the U.S. was in the May 15th 2004 issue of The Brattleboro Reformer of Brattleboro, VT. It carried an extensive article titled "Drug Offers Hope for MS Patients." It was about a man who described the improvement in his MS on LDN as "unbelievable." The article includes background information about LDN and an interview with Dr. Bihari. Every article printed is a success for the movement and enhances the snowball effect.

I imagine more press coverage will emerge after the first annual LDN Conference, which is tentatively planned for June 11th 2005 at the New York Academy of Sciences in Manhattan. The theme of the conference will be "Achieving a Clinical Trial for Low Dose Naltrexone" and Dr. Bihari will be the keynote speaker. I hope that this will happen and that it will be the first of many such conferences. All of the latest news on LDN developments can be found at the official LDN website http://www.lowdosenaltrexone.org/ which is frequently updated. My own personal website is www.marybradleybooks.com.

The internet has proved to be a remarkable tool for LDN community building. The people are passionate and they are dedicated, so I have no doubt that the drug will hit the masses. It is not a matter of if the drug will be scientifically recognized, it is a matter of when and by whom. It is not a question as to whether or not LDN works, it is a question as to how well it works. And I don't doubt that many lives will benefit from the use of LDN in the future but I cannot help but wonder exactly how many.

Just how right is Dr. Bihari? I believe that he deserves much credit and recognition that I sincerely hope he claims someday soon.